Contents

70084508

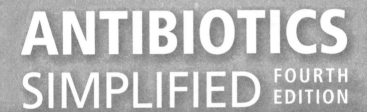

ANTIBIOTICS
SIMPLIFIED FOURTH EDITION

son C. Gallagher, PharmD, FCCP, FIDSA, BCPS
Clinical Professor
Temple University School of Pharmacy
Philadelphia, Pennsylvania

Conan MacDougall, PharmD, MAS, BCPS
Professor
University of California, San Francisco – School of Pharmacy
San Francisco, California

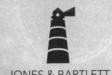

JONES & BARTLETT
LEARNING

World Headquarters
Jones & Bartlett Learning
5 Wall Street
Burlington, MA 01803
978-443-5000
info@jblearning.com
www.jblearning.com

Jones & Bartlett Learning books and products are available through most bookstores and online booksellers. To contact Jones & Bartlett Learning directly, call 800-832-0034, fax 978-443-8000, or visit our website, www.jblearning.com.

Substantial discounts on bulk quantities of Jones & Bartlett Learning publications are available to corporations, professional associations, and other qualified organizations. For details and specific discount information, contact the special sales department at Jones & Bartlett Learning via the above contact information or send an email to specialsales@jblearning.com.

The content, statements, views, and opinions herein are the sole expression of the respective authors and not that of Jones & Bartlett Learning, LLC. Reference herein to any specific commercial product, process, or service by trade name, trademark, manufacturer, or otherwise does not constitute or imply its endorsement or recommendation by Jones & Bartlett Learning, LLC and such reference shall not be used for advertising or product endorsement purposes. All trademarks displayed are the trademarks of the parties noted herein. *Antibiotics Simplified, Fourth Edition* is an independent publication and has not been authorized, sponsored, or otherwise approved by the owners of the trademarks or service marks referenced in this product.

There may be images in this book that feature models; these models do not necessarily endorse, represent, or participate in the activities represented in the images. Any screenshots in this product are for educational and instructive purposes only. Any individuals and scenarios featured in the case studies throughout this product may be real or fictitious, but are used for instructional purposes only.

The authors, editor, and publisher have made every effort to provide accurate information. However, they are not responsible for errors, omissions, or for any outcomes related to the use of the contents of this book and take no responsibility for the use of the products and procedures described. Treatments and side effects described in this book may not be applicable to all people; likewise, some people may require a dose or experience a side effect that is not described herein. Drugs and medical devices are discussed that may have limited availability controlled by the Food and Drug Administration (FDA) for use only in a research study or clinical trial. Research, clinical practice, and government regulations often change the accepted standard in this field. When consideration is being given to use of any drug in the clinical setting, the health care provider or reader is responsible for determining FDA status of the drug, reading the package insert, and reviewing prescribing information for the most up-to-date recommendations on dose, precautions, and contraindications, and determining the appropriate usage for the product. This is especially important in the case of drugs that are new or seldom used.

Production Credits

VP, Executive Publisher: David D. Cella
Publisher: Cathy L. Esperti
Editorial Assistant: Carter McAlister
Senior Vendor Manager: Sara Kelly
Associate Marketing Manager: Alianna Ortu
VP, Manufacturing and Inventory Control: Therese Connell
Composition and Project Management: Cenveo Publisher Services

Cover Design: Kristin E. Parker
Rights & Media Specialist: Jamey O'Quinn
Media Development Editor: Shannon Sheehan
Cover Image: © Triff/Shutterstock
Printing and Binding: Edwards Brothers Malloy
Cover Printing: Edwards Brothers Malloy

Library of Congress Cataloging-in-Publication Data

Names: Gallagher, Jason C., author. | MacDougall, Conan, author.
Title: Antibiotics simplified / Jason C. Gallagher, Conan MacDougall.
Description: Fourth edition. | Burlington, MA : Jones & Bartlett Learning, [2017] | Includes index.
Identifiers: LCCN 2016029350 | ISBN 9781284111293 (spiral bound : alk. paper)
Subjects: | MESH: Anti-Bacterial Agents | Handbooks
Classification: LCC RM267 | NLM QV 39 | DDC 615/.7922—dc23
LC record available at https://lccn.loc.gov/2016029350

6048

Printed in the United States of America
20 19 18 17 16   10 9 8 7 6 5 4 3 2 1

Acknowledgments

Our thanks go to those who helped edit all four editions of *Antibiotics Simplified*, and to our wives, who put up with us and took care of our kids while we wrote the *Fourth Edition*.

We dedicate this text to the pharmacy students of Temple University and University of California–San Francisco. We hope you find it useful.

Introduction

Antibiotics—the word sends terror coursing through the veins of students and makes many healthcare professionals uncomfortable. The category of antibiotics actually contains many different classes of drugs that differ in spectrum of activity, adverse effect profiles, pharmacokinetics and pharmacodynamics, and clinical utility. These classes can seem bewildering and beyond comprehension. We believe that taking a logical, stepwise approach to learning the pharmacotherapy of infectious diseases can help burn away the mental fog preventing optimal use and understanding of these drugs.

Learning the characteristics of antibiotics greatly simplifies learning infectious disease pharmacotherapy. Students and clinicians who attempt to learn the antibiotics of choice for different types of infections before knowing the characteristics of those drugs never truly understand the context of what they are attempting to learn. Once the characteristics of the antibiotics are known, making a logical choice to treat an infection is much easier. This approach takes some time up front, but it will be well worth the effort when one realizes that the pharmacotherapy of *all* infections is fundamentally similar and logical. It also pays off when you encounter a patient who didn't read the guidelines for the infection they have and requires an antibiotic regimen outside of the norm.

How to Use This Book

We wrote this book in an effort to condense the many facts that are taught about antibiotics in pharmacology and pharmacotherapy courses into one quick reference guide. It is meant to supplement material learned in pharmacology, not to supplant it. Use this book as a reference when you encounter a class of antibiotics that you know you have heard about; it will remind you of key points you may have forgotten.

This book contains six parts. Part 1 reviews basic microbiology and how to approach the pharmacotherapy of a patient with a presumed infection. The chapters in Parts 2–6 provide concise reviews of various classes of antibacterial, antimycobacterial, antifungal, antiviral, and antiparasitic drugs. Again, this book is intended to supplement your other pharmacology textbooks. These chapters give key points about each class of antibiotics—they are not thorough reviews. The appendices contain references that may help in daily use.

Format of the Drug Class Reviews

Each drug class chapter follows the same basic format. The agents belonging to each class are listed first. The drugs used most commonly in practice are in **bold**.

Mechanism of Action

This section concisely summarizes the mechanism of action of the antibiotic class.

Spectrum

This section summarizes key organisms against which each class has or lacks activity. The spectra listed are not exhaustive.

Adverse Effects

This section lists key adverse effects. This list is not exhaustive, but it gives the most common and/or concerning adverse effects of each class.

Dosing Issues

This section discusses common problems or potential errors in drug dosing for select drug classes when they are present.

Important Facts

This section provides a summary of significant facts for and aspects of each drug class.

What They're Good For

This section lists some of the most common and/or useful indications for the agents in the class. Often the agents discussed have not been approved for these indications by the U.S. Food and Drug Administration (FDA), but they are commonly used for them anyway. Conversely, many FDA indications that the antibiotics do have are not listed here, because they are often out-of-date.

Don't Forget!

In this section, we list points that are often overlooked or especially important when dealing with the drug class.

As you read this book, try to think of situations in which the antibiotics would be useful to your patients. Think of *why* an antibiotic is useful for an indication; don't just learn *that* it is. It is our sincere hope that you too have that magic moment where the world of antibiotics and the study of infectious diseases click together. Let us know when it happens.

New to the *Fourth Edition*

The *Fourth Edition* of *Antibiotics Simplified* expands on the drug classes covered in the previous editions while retaining the "key point" focus of the text that has made it successful. A new chapter—Chapter 6—has been added to Part I to (hopefully) simplify the complex nature of antibiotic resistance. The *Fourth Edition* includes expanded coverage of new agents, including the rapidly changing world of hepatitis C pharmacotherapy. New antibiotics have been added since the *Third Edition*, and the chapters for each class were updated with new clinical and scientific findings.

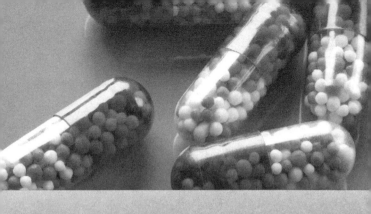

Considerations with Antibiotic Therapy

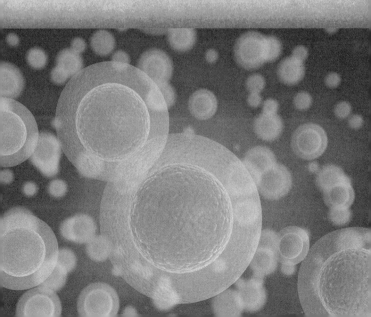

PART 1

The Wonderful World of Microbiology

Despite the promises of the household-products industry, almost *every surface* is covered in microorganisms almost *all the time*. Swab a countertop, your skin, or your dinner and you will find a little world—and that covers only the estimated 1% of bacteria that can be cultured! Obviously, trying to sterilize our patients (and our countertops) is futile; we have to try to target the bad organisms and let the rest happily crawl all over us—they greatly outnumber our own cells in our own bodies anyway.

In the microbial world, bacteria lie toward the "less like us" end of the spectrum (Figure 1-1). They are prokaryotes, not eukaryotes like fungi, protozoa, and humans. Viruses are even more different from us—they are basically just a package of genetic instructions in a cell-attacking protein coat (Figure 1-2). Differences between cells of microorganisms and humans in anatomy, biochemistry, and affinity of antibiotics for their targets are what allow for the safe and efficacious use of antibiotics. In this section we will concentrate on the microbiology of bacteria. Discussion of the unique characteristics of fungi, viruses, mycobacteria, and parasites will be covered in the sections where agents active against those organisms are introduced.

Less like us

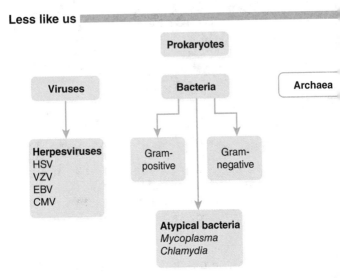

Figure 1–1
The Microbial World

Differentiating bacteria that are responsible for infection from those just along for the ride can be difficult. Many bacteria that can cause human disease are also normal commensal flora, including *Escherichia coli, Streptococcus pneumoniae,* and *Staphylococcus aureus.* Thus, growth of one of these organisms from a culture is not necessarily synonymous with infection. Suspicion of infection is increased greatly if the organism grows from a normally sterile site, such as the bloodstream or cerebrospinal fluid (CSF). Indicators of infection in nonsterile sites (such as sputum and wound cultures) are a high number of organisms, presence of inflammatory cells, and symptoms referable to

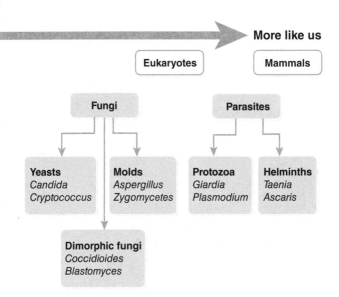

the culture site (e.g., cough or dyspnea in a patient with a sputum culture growing *S. pneumoniae*, redness and pain in a patient with a skin culture growing *S. aureus*).

Definitive identification and susceptibility testing may take anywhere from hours to months, depending on the organism and the methods used. Microscopic examination and staining may allow for rapid preliminary identification. For bacteria, the most important of these techniques is the Gram stain. Being able to interpret preliminary results of microbiology testing will allow you to provide the most appropriate therapy for your patients as early as possible.

One of the most fundamental differences among types of bacteria is how they react to a Gram stain.

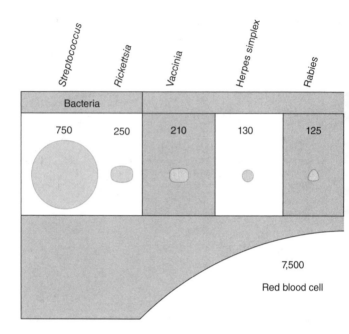

Figure 1–2
Relative Sizes of Microorganisms

Gram stain (crystal violet) is a substance that selectively stains the cell walls of Gram-positive bacteria but is easily washed away from Gram-negative bacteria. Why? In Gram-positive bacteria, the outermost membrane is a thick layer of peptidoglycan, a cellular substance that gives bacterial cells rigidity. In contrast, Gram-negative bacteria have an outer membrane of lipopolysaccharide that blocks the stain from adhering to the peptidoglycan within the cell (Figure 1–3).

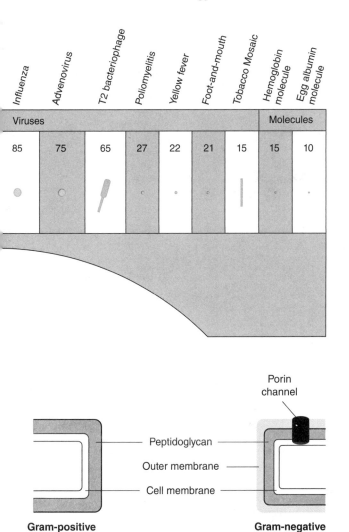

Influenza	Adenovirus	T2 bacteriophage	Poliomyelitis	Yellow fever	Foot-and-mouth	Tobacco Mosaic	Hemoglobin molecule	Egg albumin molecule
Viruses							Molecules	
85	75	65	27	22	21	15	15	10

Figure 1–3

Cell Walls of Gram-Positive and Gram-Negative Organisms

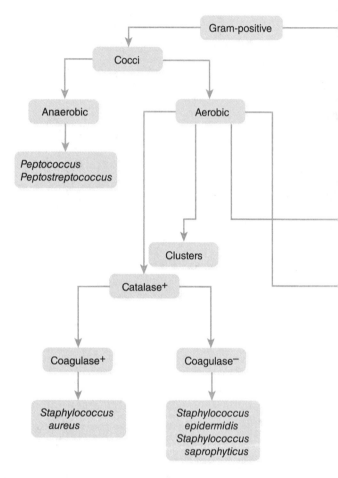

Figure 1–4
Gram-Positive Bacteria

Rapid identification of Gram-positive bacteria based on morphology and preliminary biochemical tests can help to direct therapy.

1. **Morphology:** Most medically important Gram-positive pathogens are cocci (spheres) rather than bacilli (rods). The finding of

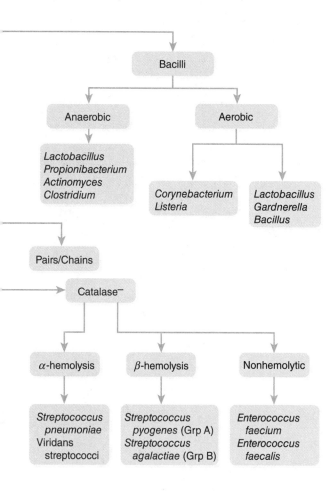

Gram-positive bacilli should be interpreted within the clinical context: in blood cultures, Gram-positive bacilli often represent common skin contaminants (such as *Propionibacterium*, *Corynebacterium*, and *Bacillus* species), since the skin barrier must be bypassed to collect the culture. Detection of Gram-positive bacilli from necrotizing wound infections suggests clostridial infection, whereas the finding of Gram-positive bacilli in CSF cultures raises the concern for *Listeria*.

2. **Colony clustering:** Within the Gram-positive cocci, the staphylococci tend to form clusters, whereas the streptococci (including enterococci) typically appear in pairs or chains. Again, the clinical context aids in interpretation: The finding of streptococci in a respiratory culture suggests *S. pneumoniae*, while a report of "streptococci" from an intra-abdominal culture suggests *Enterococcus* (which may be identified preliminarily as a *Streptococcus*).

3. **Biochemistry and appearance on agar:** The rapid catalase test helps to differentiate staphylococci from streptococci. The coagulase test is useful for differentiating the more virulent (coagulase-positive) *S. aureus* from its cousin the coagulase-negative *Staphylococcus epidermidis*. *S. epidermidis* is a frequent contaminant of blood cultures; if only one of a pair of blood samples is positive for coagulase-negative staphylococci, treatment may not be required. The pattern of hemolysis (clearing around colonies on agar plates) helps to differentiate among the streptococci: the oral flora (α-hemolytic *S. pneumoniae* and the viridans streptococci); pathogens of the skin, pharynx, and genitourinary tract (β-hemolytic Group A and β strep); and the bugs of gastrointestinal origin (nonhemolytic enterococci: the more common *Enterococcus faecalis* and the more resistant *Enterococcus faecium*).

Gram-negatives also contain peptidoglycan, but in smaller amounts, and it is not the outermost layer of the cell. Both Gram-positive and Gram-negative organisms contain an inner cell membrane that separates the cell wall from the cytoplasm of the organism.

Figures 1–4 and 1–5 show how you can identify different bacteria by differences in morphology, oxygen tolerance, and biochemical identification.

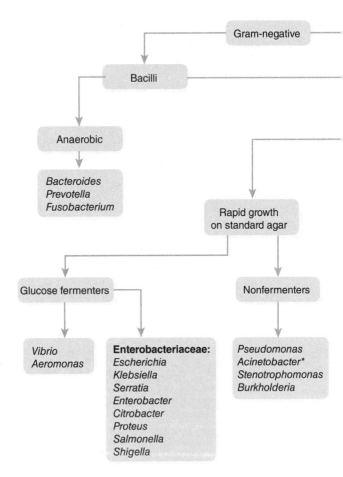

Figure 1–5
Gram-Negative Bacteria

Preliminary identification is somewhat less useful with the Gram-negative bacteria because more extensive biochemical tests are usually needed to differentiate among them.

1. **Morphology:** Among Gram-negative pathogens, the bacilli predominate. The situation in which identification of Gram-negative cocci is

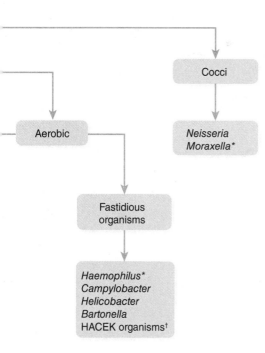

* = these organisms may appear as coccobacilli
† = *Haemophilus, Actinobacillus, Cardiobacterium, Eikenella, Kingella*

most useful is in the setting of meningitis, where this finding would strongly suggest *Neisseria meningitidis*. Note also that some organisms have an intermediate or "coccobacillary" appearance, which may suggest organisms of the genera *Haemophilus*, *Moraxella*, or *Acinetobacter*.

2. **Glucose/lactose fermentation:** The pathogens within the family Enterobacteriaceae (including *E. coli*, *Klebsiella*, *Serratia*, and *Enterobacter*) generally ferment glucose/lactose; at this point the lab may identify them as "enteric Gram-negative rods" or

"lactose-fermenting Gram-negative rods." In contrast, *Pseudomonas*, *Acinetobacter*, *Stenotrophomonas*, and *Burkholderia* are "nonfermenters"; a report of "nonfermenting Gram-negative rods" should lead you to reassess and if necessary broaden your antibiotic coverage, because many of these organisms have a high level of antibiotic resistance.

3. **Fastidious organisms:** These organisms are picky eaters—they grow slowly and often require specially supplemented media. Thus, it may take a few days to a few weeks for them to grow from culture.

General Approach to Infectious Diseases

The pharmacotherapy of infectious diseases is unique. In the pharmacotherapy of most diseases, we give drugs that have some desired pharmacologic action at some receptor or protein in the *patient*. To treat infections, we give antibiotics to exert a desired pharmacologic effect on the *organism* that is causing infection in the patient. With few exceptions, direct effects on the patients from antibiotics are not desired and are adverse effects. It is the third point in the triangle of infectious diseases pharmacotherapy, the pathogen, which makes each infection in each patient unique (Figure 2–1). The fact that the pharmacotherapy of infectious diseases involves organisms that change and "fight back" confuses many clinicians, but the approach to the patient with an infection is relatively simple and consistent. Understanding this approach is the first step in developing a useful expertise in infectious diseases and antibiotic use.

A note: technically the term *antibiotic* refers only to a subset of antibacterial drugs that are natural products. The terms *anti-infective* and *antimicrobial* encompass antibacterial, antifungal, antiviral, and antiparasitic drugs. However, because *antibiotic* is the more commonly used term, we will use it to refer to antimicrobials in general or antibacterials specifically.

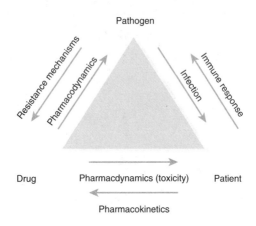

Figure 2–1
Relationships in the Infected Patient

Prophylactic Therapy

The use of antimicrobial chemotherapy—that is, the treatment of microorganisms with chemical agents—falls into one of three general categories: prophylaxis, empiric use, and definitive therapy. *Prophylaxis* is treatment given to prevent an infection that has not yet developed. Use of prophylactic therapy should be limited to patients at high risk of developing an infection, such as those on immunosuppressive therapy, those with cancer, or patients who are having surgery. These patients have weakened natural defenses that render them susceptible to infection. Because the likelihood of infection by some types of organisms in these patients is high and the consequences of infection are dire, we administer antimicrobial drugs to prevent infections from occurring. However, the world is not sterile and breakthrough infections do occur. The key to understanding antimicrobial prophylaxis is to remember that patients who receive it do not have an infection, but they are at risk for one.

Empiric Therapy

Unlike prophylactic therapy, *empiric therapy* is given to patients who have a proven or suspected infection, but the responsible organism(s) has or have not yet been identified. It is the type of therapy most often initiated in both outpatient and inpatient settings. After the clinician assesses the likelihood of an infection based on physical exam, laboratory findings, and other signs and symptoms, he or she should generally collect samples for culture and Gram staining. For most types of cultures, the Gram stain is performed relatively quickly. In the Gram stain, details about the site of presumed infection are revealed, such as the presence of organisms and white blood cells (WBCs), morphology of the organisms present (e.g., Gram-positive cocci in clusters), and the nature of the sample itself, which in some cases indicates if the sample is adequate. The process of culturing the sample begins around the time that the clinician performs the Gram stain. After a day or so, biochemical testing will reveal the identification of the organism, and eventually the organism will be tested for its susceptibility to various antibiotics.

However, this process takes several days, so empiric therapy is generally initiated *before* the clinician knows the exact identification and susceptibilities of the causative organism. Empiric therapy is our best guess of which antimicrobial agent or agents will be most active against the likely cause of infection. Sometimes we are right, and sometimes we are wrong. Keep in mind that empiric therapy should not be directed against every known organism in nature—just those most likely to cause the infection in question. In other words, broad-spectrum antibiotics are not a substitute for rational thought!

Definitive Therapy

After culture and sensitivity results are known, the *definitive therapy* phase of treatment can begin. Unlike empiric therapy, with definitive therapy we know on what organisms to base our treatment and which drugs should work against them. At this phase, it is prudent to choose antimicrobial agents that are safe, effective, narrow in spectrum, and cost effective. This helps us avoid unneeded toxicity, treatment failures, and the possible emergence of antimicrobial resistance, and it also helps manage costs. In general, moving from empiric to definitive therapy involves decreasing coverage (assuming the empiric choice ended up being correct for the organism that grew), because we do not need to target organisms that are not causing infection in our patient. In fact, giving overly broad-spectrum antibiotics can lead to the development of superinfections, infections caused by organisms resistant to the antibiotics in use that occur during therapy.

The clinician who is treating an infected patient should always strive to make the transition to definitive therapy. Although it seems obvious, this does not always occur. If the patient improves on the first antibiotic, clinicians may be reluctant to transition to more narrow-spectrum therapy. Also, some infections may resolve with empiric therapy before culture results would even be available, as frequently happens with uncomplicated urinary tract infections (UTIs). In other cases, cultures may not be obtained or may be negative in spite of strong signs that the patient has an infection (e.g., clinical symptoms, fever, increased WBC count). Outpatient clinicians frequently skip the culture collection step, begin empiric therapy, and wait to see what happens. This may be because of time pressures or the perceived cost and inconvenience of obtaining cultures in patients with low-acuity infections. In most situations it is important that clinicians continuously consider the need to transition to definitive therapy. Overly broad-spectrum therapy has consequences, and the next infection is likely to be harder to treat. Excessive empiric antibiotic use is a big part of the reason there is an antimicrobial resistance crisis. Keep in mind the general pathway for the treatment of infectious diseases shown in Figure 2–2.

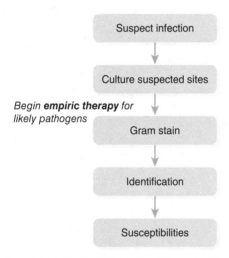

*Change to **definitive therapy** for patient-specific pathogens*

Figure 2–2
General Approach to Infectious Diseases

Examples of Therapy

Here are a few examples of each type of therapy:

Prophylaxis Therapy

- Trimethoprim/sulfamethoxazole (TMP/SMX) to prevent *Pneumocystis jirovecii* (formerly *carinii*) pneumonia in a patient on cyclosporine and prednisone after a liver transplant
- Azithromycin to prevent *Mycobacterium avium intracellularae* (MAI or MAC) in an HIV patient with a low CD4 count
- Cefazolin given before surgery to prevent a staphylococcal skin infection of the surgical site

Empiric Therapy

- Levofloxacin initiated for a patient with presumed community-acquired pneumonia
- Ceftriaxone given for the treatment of suspected pyelonephritis
- Voriconazole initiated for a neutropenic bone marrow transplant patient with shortness of breath and a radiograph suggestive of pulmonary aspergillosis
- Vancomycin, tobramycin, and meropenem for a patient with probable hospital-acquired pneumonia in the intensive care unit

Definitive Therapy

- Transitioning from piperacillin/tazobactam to ampicillin in a patient with a wound infection caused by *Enterococcus faecalis*, which is susceptible to both drugs
- Discontinuing ceftriaxone and initiating ciprofloxacin for a patient with a UTI caused

by *Klebsiella pneumoniae* that is resistant to ceftriaxone but susceptible to ciprofloxacin
- Stopping caspofungin and initiating fluconazole for an improving patient with *Candida* in a blood isolate when the species is identified as *Candida albicans* (which is generally susceptible to fluconazole)
- Narrowing therapy from vancomycin, ciprofloxacin, and imipenem/cilastatin to linezolid alone for a patient with hospital-acquired pneumonia whose deep respiratory culture grew only methicillin-resistant *Staphylococcus aureus* (MRSA) that is susceptible to linezolid

Case Study

Here is an example of treating a patient with an infection by the above pathway:

TR is a 63-year-old man with a history of diabetes, hypertension, and coronary artery disease who comes to the hospital complaining of pain, redness, and swelling around a wound on his foot. Close inspection reveals that he has an infected diabetic foot ulcer. He is admitted to the hospital (Day 1). A surgeon performs surgical debridement that evening and sends cultures from the wound during surgery as well as blood cultures. Another clinician initiates *empiric therapy* with vancomycin and ertapenem.

On Day 2, Gram stain results from the wound are available. There are many WBCs with many Gram-positive cocci in clusters but no Gram-negative rods (GNRs), so the clinician discontinues ertapenem. Blood cultures do not grow any organisms.

The following day (Day 3), culture results from the wound reveal many *Staphylococcus aureus*.

Because vancomycin is usually effective against this organism, its use is continued.

On Day 4, susceptibility results from the wound culture return. The *S. aureus* is found to be susceptible to methicillin, oxacillin, cefazolin, clindamycin, TMP/SMX, and vancomycin. It is resistant to penicillin, ampicillin, tetracycline, and levofloxacin. Because the isolate from TR's wound is methicillin-susceptible *S. aureus* (MSSA), the clinician discontinues vancomycin and initiates *definitive therapy* with oxacillin.

Note how in TR's case we began empiric therapy with a broad-spectrum regimen of vancomycin and ertapenem to cover the Gram-positive and Gram-negative aerobes and anaerobes that tend to cause diabetic foot infections but narrowed that therapy gradually as Gram stain and culture data returned. Eventually we were able to choose a highly effective, narrow-spectrum, inexpensive, and safe choice of definitive therapy that was driven by microbiology results. Both vancomycin and ertapenem were active against TR's *S. aureus* as well, but both are broader in spectrum than oxacillin and represent less-ideal therapy choices. Note: ertapenem's activity against this isolate is inferred from the susceptibility pattern even though it was not tested directly.

A Note on Rapid Diagnostics

Slowly, novel ways to determine the identification of microorganisms are making their way into clinical practice. Techniques that do not rely on culturing and the inherent delay that it represents are already commonly used to detect and quantify many viruses, such as polymerase chain reactions (PCR). These and other techniques are being used to identify other pathogens as well, such as strains of *Candida* (to determine likely fluconazole susceptibility), *Clostridium difficile*, and even MRSA. As they permeate clinical microbiology labs, hopefully the delays to effective therapy that current gold-standard culture and susceptibility testing cause will vanish.

Antibiotic Pharmacokinetics

3

The term *antibiotic pharmacokinetics* refers to *how* (and to *what extent*) antibiotics *enter the body*, *where they go* once they are "inside," and *how they get out*. These three phases of pharmacokinetics are usually described as *absorption*, *distribution*, and *metabolism / excretion* (sometimes abbreviated "ADME"). The pharmacokinetics of antibiotics are key to the effectiveness of the drugs in clinical practice; there is no benefit for a patient to receive an antibiotic that is great at killing bugs if it never gets to the site of the infection at a high enough concentration to work. If you think about it, this is an issue for most types of human disease, but in infectious diseases it is very relevant clinically. You don't have to wonder if phenytoin distributes to the central nervous system (CNS)—it does, or else it would be worthless for seizures. However, it is important to know that ceftriaxone distributes there well but cefazolin does not if you are treating meningitis. Figure 3–1 illustrates ADME phases on a concentration–time curve, with the concentration of the drug on the Y axis and the time since drug administration on the X axis. It also indicates the key pharmacokinetic parameters of peak concentration, trough concentration, and area under the concentration–time curve ("AUC").

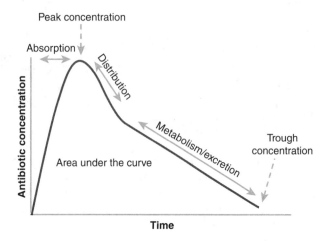

Figure 3–1
Pharmacokinetic Phases and Parameters

Absorption

Although the term "absorption" can be applied to any route of administration (e.g., absorption from intramuscular injection or inhalation), usually it is used to refer to the uptake of orally administered drugs into the bloodstream. The percentage of a nonintravenously administered drug that enters the bloodstream (such as an oral drug), relative to an intravenous formulation of the same drug, is termed the *bioavailability*. Antibiotics with oral formulations differ substantially in their bioavailability. For some antibiotics, bioavailability is at or near 100%; the same dose administered orally or intravenously will achieve similar levels. It is worth considering that several antibiotics have very good bioavailability, but their oral doses are substantially lower than the intravenous doses. This is usually because high oral doses lead to excessive gastrointestinal (GI) tract toxicity. Table 3–1 groups antibiotics into groups with high oral bioavailability and full or near intravenous–oral dose equivalence, those with good oral bioavailability but substantially lower oral than intravenous doses, and those with limited oral bioavailability. Some oral antibiotics have almost zero bioavailability and take advantage of this clinically to eradicate pathogens in the GI tract, where they achieve much higher concentrations than they would if given intravenously.

TABLE 3–1

Examples of Absorption for Different Oral Antibiotics

Drug	Bioavailability	Typical Intravenous Dose	Typical Oral Dose
Drugs with High Bioavailability and Similar Intravenous–Oral Doses			
Metronidazole	95–100%	500 mg IV q8h	500 mg PO q8h
Levofloxacin	95–100%	500–750 mg IV q24h	500–750 mg PO daily
Linezolid	95–100%	600 mg IV q8h	600 mg PO q12h
Fluconazole	95–100%	200–400 mg IV daily	200–400 mg PO daily
Doxycycline	95–100%	100 mg IV q12h	100 mg PO q12h
Ciprofloxacin	~80%	400 mg IV q12h	500 mg PO q12h
Drugs with High Bioavailability but Different Intravenous–Oral Doses			
Aminopenicillins	~90%	Ampicillin: 1–2 g IV q4–6h	Amoxicillin: 500 mg–1 g PO TID
First-generation cephalosporins	~90%	Cefazolin: 1–2 g IV q8h	Cephalexin: 500 mg PO QID
Drugs with Low Bioavailability and Different Intravenous–Oral Doses			
Cefuroxime	~40%	750 mg IV q8h	500 mg PO BID
Acyclovir	~25%	5 mg/kg IV q8h	400 mg PO TID

It is important to consider factors that can affect the bioavailability of antibiotics. Three factors that can substantially influence absorption are food, gastric acidity, and chelating agents. Some antibiotics are better absorbed with food and some without, while for most antibiotics the presence or absence of food has minimal effect.

A small group of antibiotics are highly dependent on gastric acidity for adequate absorption; it is important to avoid concomitant use of drugs that raise gastric pH (antacids, proton pump inhibitors, histamine-2 receptor antagonists) when patients are started on these drugs. Finally, two key classes of antibiotics—the tetracyclines and fluoroquinolones—can bind to coadministered minerals present in the gut such as calcium, iron, aluminum, and zinc. Administering these drugs along with mineral or some vitamin supplements can substantially reduce absorption. Table 3–2 provides examples of antibiotics where these factors need to be accounted for.

TABLE 3–2

Examples of Antibiotics Whose Absorption Is Significantly Affected by Other Factors

Absorption Improved with Food	Absorption Impaired by Food	Absorption Impaired by Drugs That Increase Gastric pH	Absorption Impaired by Minerals
Posaconazole suspension	Voriconazole	Itraconazole	Fluoroquinolones
Itraconazole capsules	Itraconazole solution	Posaconazole suspension	Tetracyclines
Atazanavir	Rifampin	Atazanavir	
Darunavir	Isoniazid	Rilpivirine	
Rilpivirine	Pyrazinamide		

Distribution

After a drug is absorbed or injected into the blood-stream, it moves into various tissues (e.g., bone, cerebrospinal fluid, lungs), a process known as *distribution*. The concentrations in these tissues can be similar to, lower than, or greater than the concentration of the antibiotic in the blood. A consequence is that a drug may be more or less effective in a particular tissue than would be expected based on its concentrations in the blood. For example, the concentrations of antibiotics in the cerebrospinal fluid are typically much lower than their blood-stream concentrations, limiting the effectiveness of many antibiotics in the treatment of meningitis. On the other hand, the macrolide antibiotics are more effective in lung infections than may be anticipated based on their blood levels, because they concentrate in pulmonary macrophages. With a few exceptions such as cerebrospinal fluid, it is difficult to obtain samples of human tissues to determine antibiotic concentrations, and it is technically difficult to measure the concentrations in tissues like bone. Thus, data on drug distribution are often extrapolated from animal models, which may or may not be good surrogates for humans.

The extent to which antibiotics distribute into different tissues is largely determined by the physicochemical properties of the drug (lipophilicity, charge, molecular size, etc.). A key determinant of distribution is the degree to which an antibiotic binds to proteins in the bloodstream, most importantly albumin (you may hear this expressed as "fraction bound" or "fraction unbound"). Drug bound to proteins is not able to diffuse across membranes into different tissues; thus, antibiotics that are highly protein bound *may* be less likely to reach effective concentrations in certain tissues (such as the CNS). It is important to realize that the percentage degree of penetration of an antibiotic into a tissue is not the only determinant of effectiveness in that tissue. For example, ceftriaxone is a very highly protein-bound drug, and 5% or less enters into the CNS in patients with meningitis. However, large doses (2 g twice daily in adults) of ceftriaxone can be given safely to adults, resulting in high serum levels (peak levels of around 200 mg/L). In addition, the minimum inhibitory concentration (MIC) to ceftriaxone for organisms usually causing meningitis is typically very low (1 mg/L or less); thus, a concentration far in excess of the organism's MIC can be obtained (200 mg/L × 5% = 10 mg/L). Also, the concentration–time curves in many tissues are different than they are in the bloodstream—more like rolling hills than peaks and valleys (think Appalachians versus the Rockies).

Patient characteristics may also significantly influence drug distribution. In order for a drug to distribute to a tissue, there must be adequate blood flow to that tissue. Conditions that reduce blood flow to tissues, either locally (e.g., peripheral vascular disease) or systemically (septic shock), can reduce antibiotic concentrations at the site of infection. Patients with severe infections can develop abscesses or areas of dead and devitalized tissue; distribution of antibiotics into these "protected" sites of infection can be significantly impaired. These patients are perfect setups for treatment failure and development of resistance and highlight the importance of appropriate surgical management of infections along with antibiotic treatment. Given the growing problem of obesity, another important consideration is the extent to which drugs distribute into adipose tissue. Depending on the characteristics of the drug, it is possible to underdose patients who are morbidly obese (if the drug distributes extensively into adipose tissue and doses for standard weights are used) or overdose them (if a higher dose is used because of obesity, but the drug does not distribute well into excess adipose tissue). Thus, you may see recommendations for antibiotic dosing based on *total or actual* body weight, *ideal* body weight (an estimate of the patient's body weight without their excess adipose tissue), or *adjusted* body weight (a value between the ideal and total body weight). This is an area that is relatively understudied.

Finally, it is important to note that with few exceptions, microbiological susceptibility testing does not account for distribution and is based on achievable bloodstream concentrations. For example, the microbiology lab may determine that an organism with an MIC of 4 mg/L is considered susceptible to a drug that achieves a concentration of 8 mg/L in the bloodstream, but it may only achieve a concentration of 1 mg/L in cerebrospinal fluid. Thus, that drug is likely to work for a bloodstream infection caused by the organism, but would fail for meningitis where cerebrospinal fluid concentrations are important. Thus, distribution is a key consideration when choosing antibiotics.

Metabolism/Excretion

Many antibiotics are excreted from the body, either in the urine or feces, in the same form as they were administered. In fact, shortly after penicillin was developed and supplies were scarce, doctors used to collect the urine of patients who received penicillin and recrystallize the drug for use in other patients! When a drug is excreted unchanged, it can reach very high concentrations in the area in which it is eliminated, making it potentially more effective for infections in those systems than would be anticipated based on blood concentrations. For example, the concentrations of nitrofurantoin achieved in the blood and tissues are generally inadequate to inhibit bacterial growth. However, it is removed from the bloodstream by the kidneys and accumulates in the bladder until its, ahem, final clearance. The concentrations achieved in the bladder are manyfold higher than those in the bloodstream, making nitrofurantoin an effective drug for treatment of bladder infections.

When the body does not inactivate the drug, an important consideration is to appropriately reduce the administered dose of the drug if there is damage to the organ responsible for excreting the drug. The most common example of this for antibiotics is the need to reduce the doses of most beta-lactams for patients with kidney dysfunction to avoid accumulation of toxic levels of the drug. Practitioners also need to be vigilant to increase doses if patients have improving renal function or treatment failure may occur.

Other drugs may be extensively transformed by the body prior to their excretion. These antibiotics that undergo extensive metabolism are considered to be *substrates* of drug-metabolizing enzymes. They have the potential to be subject to clinically important drug interactions, as other drugs may interfere with the enzymes that break the drugs down.

Moreover, certain antibiotics have the potential to influence the metabolism of other drugs, either through *inhibition* of those enzymes (leading to a decrease in metabolism of the other drug) or *induction* (leading to an increase in metabolism of the other drug). A list of antibiotics with the greatest likelihood of clinically significant metabolic drug interactions is in Table 3–3, organized by whether the drug is a substrate, an inhibitor, or an inducer (and note that drugs may be in more than one category). Note that the several antibiotic classes are particularly prevalent: macrolides, azole antifungals, antituberculosis drugs, and antiretrovirals account for most of the antibiotics with significant drug interactions. Complex drug interactions can occur with these drugs: for example, the antiretroviral drug etravirine is simultaneously a substrate, an inhibitor, and an inducer of drug-metabolizing enzymes!

TABLE 3–3

Examples of Antibiotics with Significant Metabolic Drug Interactions

Substrates	Inhibitors	Inducers
Erythromycin	TMP/SMX	Rifampin
Clarithromycin	Metronidazole	Rifabutin
Telithromycin	Fluconazole	Efavirenz
Atazanavir	Voriconazole	Nevirapine
Darunavir	Itraconazole	Etravirine
Efavirenz	Posaconazole	
Elvitegravir	Erythromycin	
Maraviroc	Clarithromycin	
Rilpivirine	Telithromycin	
	Ritonavir	
	Cobicistat	
	Etravirine	

Antibiotic Pharmacodynamics

4

The term *antibiotic pharmacodynamics* refers to the manner in which antibiotics interact with their target organisms to exert their effects: Does the antibiotic kill the organism or just prevent its growth? Is it better to give a high dose of antibiotics all at once or to achieve lower concentrations for a longer time? Clinicians increasingly recognize such considerations as important in maximizing the success of therapy, especially for difficult-to-treat infections and in immunocompromised patients.

Susceptibility Testing

Typically, one judges the susceptibility of a particular organism to an antibiotic based on the minimum inhibitory concentration (MIC) for the organism–antibiotic combination. Classically, the microbiology laboratory determines the MIC by combining a standard concentration of the organism that the patient has grown with increasing concentrations of the antibiotic. Historically this was done in test tubes (Figure 4–1), but today it is done more commonly on microdilution plates or with automated systems. The mixture is incubated for about a day, and the laboratory technician examines the tubes or plates (with the naked eye or with a computer) for signs of cloudiness, indicating

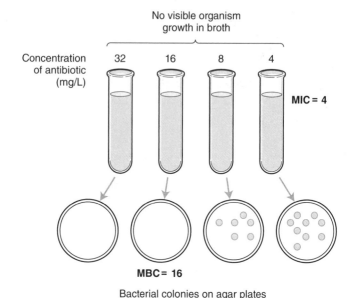

No visible organism
growth in broth

Concentration
of antibiotic
(mg/L)

32   16   8   4

MIC = 4

MBC = 16

Bacterial colonies on agar plates

Figure 4–1
Susceptibility Testing of Antibiotics

growth of the organism. The mixture with the lowest concentration of antibiotic where there is no visible growth is deemed to be the MIC. For each organism–antibiotic pair, there is a particular cutoff MIC that defines susceptibility. This particular MIC is called the *breakpoint*. Table 4–1 provides examples of how breakpoints differ for various organism/pathogen combinations and even based on the site of infection. Note that just because an antibiotic has the lowest MIC for a pathogen it does not mean it is the best choice—different antibiotics achieve different concentrations in the body in different places. Thus, antibiotic MICs for a single

Visible organism
growth in broth

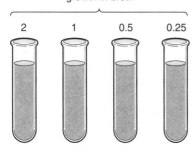

2   1   0.5   0.25

TABLE 4–1

Examples of Antibiotic Susceptibility Breakpoints

Organism Antibiotics	Susceptible (Breakpoint)	Suscep-tible, Dose-Dependent	Intermediate	Resistant
Escherichia Coli				
Ampicillin	≤ 8 mg/L	—	16 mg/L	≥ 32 mg/L
Cefepime	≤ 2 mg/L	4–8 mg/L	—	≥16 mg/L
Levofloxacin	≤ 2 mg/L	—	4 mg/L	≥ 8 mg/L
Trimethoprim/sulfamethox-azole	≤ 2/38 mg/L	—	—	≥ 4/76 mg/L
Streptococcus pneumoniae				
Ampicillin	—	—	—	—
Cefepime (meningitis)	≤ 0.5 mg/L	—	1 mg/L	≥2 mg/L
(Nonmenin-geal)	≤ 1 mg/L	—	2 mg/L	≥ 4 mg/L
Levofloxacin	≤ 2 mg/L	—	4 mg/L	≥ 8 mg/L
Trimethoprim/sulfamethox-azole	≤ 0.5/9.5 mg/L	—	1–2/19–38 mg/L	≥ 4/76 mg/L

organism generally should not be compared across different drugs in selecting therapy.

MIC values are often misinterpreted by clinicians who are trying to choose the best therapy for their patients but may inadvertently ignore pharmacokinetic and pharmacodynamic differences between agents. For example, in Table 4–1, note that the breakpoint for levofloxacin against *Escherichia coli* is 2 mg/L and for ampicillin 8 mg/L. So if an isolate of *E. coli* in the bloodstream of a patient has an MIC of 1 mg/L to levofloxacin but 2 mg/L to ampicillin, it does not mean that levofloxacin is a better choice for that patient. Levofloxacin is a concentration-dependent drug that is typically dosed in amounts of 500–750 mg daily. Ampicillin is a time-dependent drug that is typically dosed as 1–2 g every 4–6 hours. The much higher concentrations of ampicillin achieved in the body (due to higher doses) mean that organisms with a higher MIC to ampicillin are still susceptible to it. In other words, the two numbers are not directly comparable. In fact, if the MIC was 8 mg/L to both drugs, the organism would be considered resistant to levofloxacin and susceptible to ampicillin.

Also note in Table 4–1 the categories of "susceptible," "susceptible, dose-dependent," "intermediate," and "resistant." "Susceptible" and "resistant" are self-explanatory, but what do the other terms mean? "Intermediate" is a poorly defined range where successful therapy may be possible in some circumstances, such as when the drug is eliminated renally (for a urinary tract infection) or if higher dosing is given. It is more of a grey area made to separate the two more definitive terms than a scientifically derived definition. "Susceptible, dose-dependent" is just what it sounds like—the organism may be susceptible to high doses of the drug, but is likely to be resistant to low doses. This was created because many of these drugs are used in various doses, and a low dose of cefepime like 1 g IV q12h may be enough to treat an *E. coli* infection with an MIC of 2 mg/L, but a dose like 2 g IV q12h may be needed if the MIC is 4 mg/L. These may all sound like hard-and-fast rules, but they are really probabilities of how *most patients* will fare when faced with a certain bug–drug combination for their infections. Some will succeed even with high MICs, and some will fail even with low ones.

Finally, be aware that other methods of susceptibility testing exist, including disk diffusion and E-tests, but that broth dilution methods are generally considered the gold standard.

Static Versus Cidal

At the MIC the antibiotic is inhibiting growth, but it may or may not actually be killing the organism. Antibiotics that inhibit growth of the organism without killing it are termed *bacteriostatic* (or *fungistatic* in the case of fungi). If antibiotics are removed, the organisms can begin growing again. However, bacteriostatic antibiotics are usually successful in treating infections because they allow the patient's immune system to "catch up" and kill off the organisms. Other antibiotics are considered *bactericidal*; their action kills the organisms without any help from the immune system.

For most infections, outcomes using appropriate bacteriostatic versus bactericidal drugs are similar; however, for certain infections bactericidal drugs are preferred. Such infections include endocarditis, meningitis, infections in neutropenic patients, and possibly osteomyelitis. The immune system may not be as effective in fighting these infections because of the anatomic location or the immunosuppression of the patient. Bactericidal activity is determined by taking a sample of the broth at various concentrations and below and spreading the broth on agar plates (Figure 4–1). The bacterial colonies on the plates are counted, and the concentration corresponding to a 99.9% reduction (3-log) in the original bacterial inoculum is considered to be the minimum bactericidal concentration (MBC). When the MBC is four times or less than the MIC, the drug is considered to be bactericidal; if the MBC/MIC ratio is greater than four, it is considered bacteriostatic. MIC testing is standard in most laboratories; MBC testing is more difficult and is not commonly done in clinical practice. Table 4–2 lists drugs and indicates whether they are generally considered bacteriostatic or bactericidal; however, it should be noted that this activity can vary based on the pathogen being treated, the achievable dose, and the growth phase of the organism.

Pharmacokinetic/Pharmacodynamic Relationships

Besides differing in whether they kill microorganisms or merely inhibit their growth, antibiotics also differ in how they manifest their effects over time. Careful studies have revealed that for certain antibiotics, activity against microorganisms correlates

TABLE 4–2
Antibiotic Pharmacodynamic Parameters

Antibiotic Class	Cidal or Static	Predictive PK/PD Parameter
Penicillins	Bactericidal	Time > MIC
Cephalosporins		
Carbapenems		
Monobactams		
Vancomycin	Bactericidal (slowly)	AUC/MIC
Fluoroquinolones	Bactericidal	Peak: MIC
Aminoglycosides		
Metronidazole		
Daptomycin		
Macrolides	Bacteriostatic	AUC/MIC
Tetracyclines		
Linezolid		

with the duration of time that the concentration of the drug remains above the MIC (time-dependent activity). For other antibiotics, antibacterial activity correlates not with the time above the MIC but with the ratio of the peak concentration of the drug to the MIC (concentration-dependent or time-independent activity). For some antibiotics, the best predictor of activity is the ratio of the area under the concentration–time curve (AUC) to the MIC. Figure 4–2 illustrates these pharmacokinetic/pharmacodynamic (PK/PD) parameters schematically, and Table 4–2 shows which parameter is most predictive of efficacy for antibiotic classes. The practical implications of these findings are in the design of antibiotic dosing schedules: aminoglycosides are now frequently given as a single large dose daily to leverage the concentration-dependent activity, while some clinicians are administering beta-lactam drugs such as ceftazidime as continuous or prolonged infusions because of their time-dependent activity. As target values for these parameters that predict efficacy are found, there may be an increase in the individualization of dosing of antibiotics to achieve these target values.

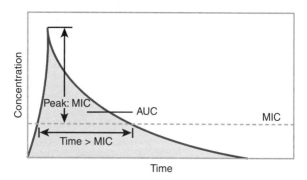

Figure 4–2
Pharmacokinetic/Pharmacodynamic Relationships

Although antibiotics are undoubtedly one of the most beneficial discoveries of science, their use does carry risks. They can adversely affect patients by eliciting allergic reactions, causing direct toxicity, or altering the normal bacterial flora, leading to superinfections with other organisms. Antibiotic use is the primary driving force in the development of antibiotic resistance, which can affect not only the treated patients but other patients by transmission of resistant organisms. It is important to keep in mind all of these potential adverse consequences when using antibiotics.

Antibiotic Allergy

Through formation of complexes with human proteins, antibiotics can trigger immunologic reactions. These reactions may manifest immediately (such as anaphylaxis or hives) or be delayed (rashes, serum sickness, drug fever). Because of their highly reactive chemical structure and frequent use, beta-lactam drugs are the most notorious group of drugs for causing allergic reactions. It is difficult to determine how likely it is that a patient with an allergy to a particular antibiotic agent will have a similar reaction to another agent within that class. While some (highly debated) estimates of the degree of cross-reactivity are available for beta-lactam drugs, estimates for cross-reactivity within other classes (e.g., between fluoroquinolones) are essentially nonexistent. Because labeling a patient with an allergy to a particular antibiotic can limit *future* treatment options severely and possibly lead to the selection of inferior drugs, every effort should be made to clarify the exact nature of a reported allergy.

Antibiotic Toxicities

Despite being designed to affect the physiology of microorganisms rather than humans, antibiotics can have direct toxic effects on patients. In some cases, this is an extension of their mechanism of action when selectivity for microorganisms is not perfect. For example, the hematologic adverse effects of trimethoprim stem from its inhibition of folate metabolism in humans, which is also its mechanism of antibiotic effect. In other cases, antibiotics display toxicity through unintended physiologic interactions, such as when vancomycin stimulates histamine release, leading to its characteristic red man syndrome. Some of these toxicities may be dose related and toxicity often occurs when doses are not adjusted properly for renal dysfunction and thus accumulate to a toxic level. Proper dosage adjustment can reduce the risk of dose-related toxicities.

Superinfection

The human body is colonized by a variety of bacteria and fungi. These organisms are generally considered commensals, in that they benefit from living on or in the body but do not cause harm (within their ecologic niches). Colonization with commensal organisms can be beneficial, given that they compete with and crowd out more pathogenic organisms. They may even have a role in the prevention of other human diseases. When administration of antibiotics kills off the commensal flora, pathogenic drug-resistant organisms can flourish because of the absence of competition. This is considered a superinfection (i.e., an infection on top of another infection). For example, administration of antibiotics can lead to the overgrowth of the gastrointestinal (GI) pathogen *Clostridium difficile*, which is clinically resistant to most antibiotics. *C. difficile* can cause diarrhea and life-threatening bowel inflammation. Similarly, administration of broad-spectrum antibacterial drugs can select for the overgrowth of fungi, most commonly yeasts of the genus *Candida*. Disseminated *Candida* infections carry a high risk of death. To reduce the risk of the impact of antibiotics on the commensal flora, and thus the likelihood of superinfection, antibiotics should be administered only to patients with proven or probable infections, using the most narrow-spectrum agents appropriate to the infection for the shortest effective duration.

Antibiotic Resistance

Thousands of studies have documented the relationship between antibiotic use and resistance, both at a patient level (if you receive an antibiotic, you are more likely to become infected with a drug-resistant organism) and a society level (the more antibiotics a hospital, region, or country uses, the greater the antibiotic resistance). The development of antibiotic resistance leads to a vicious spiral where resistance necessitates the development of broader-spectrum antibiotics, leading to evolution of bacteria resistant to those new antibiotics, requiring ever broader-spectrum drugs, and so on. This is particularly problematic because antibiotic development has slowed down greatly. Although we can see clearly the broad relationship between antibiotic use and resistance, many of the details of this relationship are not clear. Why do some bacteria develop resistance rapidly and others never develop resistance? What is the proper duration of treatment to maximize the chance of cure and minimize the risk of resistance?

6

Antibiotic Resistance

Though it may seem that the antibiotic era was introduced in the 1930s with the sulfonamides and penicillin, it had actually started millions of years earlier. Alexander Fleming only discovered one of the weapons of a war going on underfoot—literally, under our feet. In the soil and elsewhere, microbes are locked in life-and-death battles for dominance over each other for the limited resources they have access to. Among their weapons are antibiotics.

Causes of Antibiotic Resistance

The basic cause of antibiotic resistance is simple: antibiotic use. Some organisms are notorious for an intrinsic ability to express multiple types of resistance, such as *Acinetobacter baumannii* or *Pseudomonas aeruginosa*. Others have been generally treatable for many years and are only recently becoming highly drug-resistant through acquiring new resistance elements, such as *Klebsiella pneumoniae*. And some have remained highly susceptible to "old" antibiotics ever since their introduction, such as *Streptococcus pyogenes* and penicillin.

Where Does Antibiotic Resistance Come From?

In any species of bacteria, antibiotic resistance needs to have a point of origin. Resistance can emerge in the organism of interest through random mutations to the antibiotic's target or other key elements. However, it is more common that a given species of bacteria acquired the genes, which enable a mechanism of resistance, from another species of bacteria that already had it through the transfer of mobile genetic elements. Bacteria are promiscuous little organisms and they are not picky—they often swap genes not only between their own species, but different species and even genera. There are several ways that genes are transmitted between bacteria, but the most important is by the transmission of plasmids via conjugation. Plasmids are loops of DNA that may contain multiple genes in them that encode for various processes (including antibiotic resistance), and they are highly portable. Since plasmids can contain multiple genes, they can encode for multiple types of resistance that are not related, such as resistance to cephalosporins via the production of a beta-lactamase and resistance to fluoroquinolone due to an efflux pump. With one act of gene swapping, a multiply-resistant bacterial strain is born.

Mechanisms of Antibiotic Resistance

The multiple mechanisms by which resistance occurs can be confusing, but here we are going to—wait for it—simplify it into four basic mechanisms, which are outlined in Figure 6–1.

Decreased permeability prevents the antibiotic from penetrating the bacterial cell, decreasing the intracellular concentration of the antibiotic.

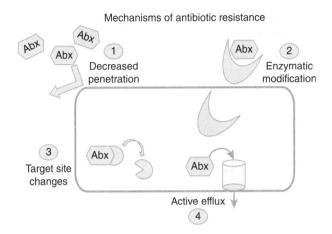

Figure 6–1
Mechanisms of Antibiotic Resistance

Enzymatic modification due to an enzyme produced by the bacteria destroys the antibiotic before it has a chance to reach its site of activity or even enter the cell. *Target site changes* can occur, leading to an elimination or modification of the antibiotic's site of activity such that it cannot work. *Active efflux* occurs when efflux pumps in the bacteria pump out antibiotics, decreasing intracellular concentrations. Examples of how common mechanisms of resistance fall into these four broad categories are given in Table 6–1.

Knowing the mechanism of resistance for a particular bug–drug combination is not essential in most clinical situations. Multiple mechanisms of resistance are often present and being expressed simultaneously, which make it impossible to infer the mechanism of resistance just from the reported

TABLE 6–1
Examples of Mechanisms of Antibiotic Resistance

Category	Example
Decreased permeability	Cell wall changes
	Porin channel changes or loss
	Biofilm production
Enzymatic modification	Beta-lactamases (over 1400 different types!)
	Aminoglycoside-modifying enzymes
	Methylation
Target site changes	PBP 2a expression in *Staphylococcus aureus*
	PBP 2x expression in *Streptococcus pneumoniae*
	Ribosomal modification
Active efflux	Tetracycline efflux
	Fluoroquinolone efflux

sensitivities. We have highlighted situations where it is more important throughout the antibacterial chapters in this text.

Antibiotic Pressure and Collateral Damage

Antibiotic use has consequences. Antibiotics are the only class of drug for which their use in one person affects their utility in another person, since microorganisms are transmissible. *Antibiotic pressure* is a term that reflects the fact that antibiotic-resistant strains may emerge when antibiotic-susceptible strains are killed. If a patient is infected or colonized with resistant and susceptible strains of a bacteria, the use of an antibiotic will kill the susceptible strain and allow the resistant one to grow. This pressure is worth the trade-off when the patient has an infection and requires treatment, but excessive pressure placed on the microorganisms in the patient can be limited by how we use antibiotics. *Collateral damage* is a term used to describe the impact of antibiotic use on microorganisms in the body beyond the targeted organism. Every dose of antibiotics affects not just the pathogen causing an infection, but billions of other bacteria in and on the body, bacteria that are just minding their business and often helping us out by preventing colonization by more aggressive bacteria. Collateral damage will occur with any antibiotic, but can be minimized by using less-broad-spectrum antibiotics and, perhaps most importantly, minimizing the duration of use of all antibiotics when possible. One of the greatest concerns and most contentious issues in antibiotic resistance is the use of antibiotics in agriculture, which is where most antibiotics in the United States are used. The impact of this and the collateral damage that it has on the human microbiome is just beginning to be determined.

The ESKAPE Pathogens

Antibiotic resistance has been described in most bacteria that cause human infection, but some pathogens are particularly problematic. There have been several ways to describe the most serious antibiotic-resistance threats that plague mankind, but probably the most commonly utilized one is the acronym "ESKAPE" (Table 6–2).

These diverse organisms have in common both, a high propensity for antibiotic resistance and limited options for treating their resistant phenotypes. The Centers for Disease Control and Prevention (CDC) published a report in 2013 titled "Antibiotic Resistance Threats in the United States, 2013"

TABLE 6–2	
"ESKAPE" Pathogens and Other Resistance Threats	
"ESKAPE" pathogens	*Enterococcus faecium*
	Staphylococcus aureus
	Klebsiella pneumoniae
	Acinetobacter baumannii
	Pseudomonas aeruginosa
	Enterobacter species
Organisms classified by CDC as an urgent health threat	*Clostridium difficile*
	Carbapenem-resistant Enterobacteriaceae
	Drug-resistant *Neisseria gonorrhoeae*

that details the estimated threat of resistance in the United States, available at http://www.cdc.gov. It estimated that 23,000 people in the United States die each year due to resistant bacterial infections, but that figure did not include the estimated 14,000 deaths per year from *C. difficile* infection.

Preventing Antibiotic Resistance—A Problem of Perspective

With all of this good news, what can we do to prevent antibiotic resistance? Convincing data show that limiting antibiotic use limits antibiotic resistance. This has been shown on many levels, from the patient- to the hospital- to the country-level. Unfortunately, each of these levels has a different perspective. Patients want to get better and may not know that the antibiotic they are requesting is unlikely to work for a viral respiratory infection. Hospitals are concerned with both patient outcomes and costs, and diagnostic uncertainty drives much empiric antibiotic use. Many clinicians are afraid to miss a potential infection and end up using antibiotics for patients who actually are not infected. Only the societal viewpoint is high-level enough to really look at overall antibiotic use and how it impacts antibiotic resistance.

Guidelines

Decisions to use antibiotics are not made by society; they are made on a patient basis. It falls upon all of us to make therapy decisions with antibiotic resistance in mind. Some general guidance for utilizing antibiotics follows below.

Avoid Using Antibiotics to Treat Colonization or Contamination

A substantial percentage of all antibiotic use is directed toward patients who are not truly infected, but in whom organisms are recovered from culture. Isolation of *Staphylococcus epidermidis* from a single blood culture or *Candida* species from a urinary culture in a catheterized patient are common situations in which patients should be scrutinized to determine whether an infection is truly present. Diagnostic improvements need to be developed and utilized when they are available. A simple test that could distinguish a cold from a bacterial infection could save society billions in avoided antibiotic use, resistance, and adverse effects.

Use the Most Narrow-Spectrum Agent Appropriate for the Patient's Infection

Broader-spectrum agents multiply the number of bacteria affected by the drug, increasing the chances both for development of resistance and superinfection. "Broader" and "newer" are not synonymous with "better": for example, good old penicillin kills susceptible organisms more rapidly than almost any drug on the market. The treating clinician's goal always should be definitive, narrow-spectrum therapy.

Use the Proper Dose

Bacteria that are exposed to low concentrations of antibiotics are more likely to become resistant than those exposed to effective doses. After all, dead bugs don't mutate! Further research in pharmacodynamics should make it easier to determine the proper dose for each patient and thus to reduce the likelihood that resistance will develop.

Use the Shortest Effective Duration of Therapy

Unfortunately, duration of therapy is one of the least-studied areas of infectious diseases. Examination of standard treatment durations says much more about how humans think than about how antibiotics and bacteria truly interact—durations are typically 5, 7, 10, or 14 days, more in line with our decimal system and the days in a week than with anything studied precisely. New studies are showing that shorter durations of therapy are often just as effective as prolonged courses and possibly less likely to select for resistance. As studies progress and determine additional factors that indicate when infections are sufficiently treated, it should be possible to define more accurately the length of therapy on a patient-by-patient basis. Many clinicians find that "old habits die hard," however, they should remember that learning new evidence about duration of therapy is important as it emerges.

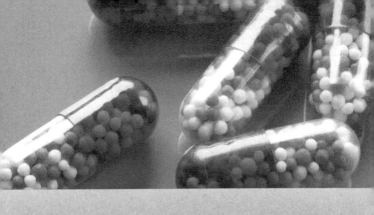

Antibacterial Drugs

PART 2

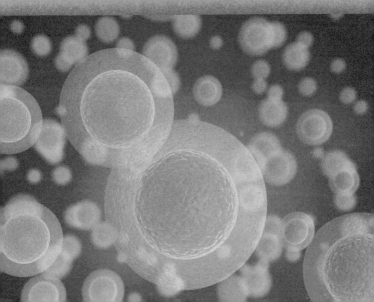

7

Beta-Lactams

Introduction to Beta-Lactams

Beta-lactams include a wide variety of antibiotics that seem to exist only to confuse both students and clinicians. Penicillins, cephalosporins, and carbapenems are all beta-lactams. Monobactams (aztreonam) are structurally similar, but they lack one of the two rings that other beta-lactams have and have little to no cross-allergenicity with other beta-lactams. To make matters more confusing, not all beta-lactams end in *-cillin* or *-penem* or start with *ceph-*.

We believe the best approach to keeping beta-lactams straight is to group them into classes and learn the characteristics of each class. If you work in a hospital, you will likely have only one or two drugs of each class to worry about. In the outpatient setting, you will encounter many more of them. Fortunately, all beta-lactams have a few things in common:

- All beta-lactams can cause hypersensitivity reactions, ranging from mild rashes to drug fever to acute interstitial nephritis (AIN) to anaphylaxis. There is some cross-sensitivity among classes, but there is no way to predict exactly how often that will occur. Studies on the matter differ greatly in their conclusions, though on the whole cross-sensitivity seems to be lower between different types of beta-lactams than previously thought. There is an evolving school of thought that the similarities between side chains of beta-lactams are responsible for cross-sensitivity and that the likelihood of allergic reactions can be predicted by them, but this has not disseminated widely into clinical practice.

- Seizures can result from very high doses of any beta-lactam, and some cause other neurologic effects. Accumulation to toxic levels can occur when the dose of a beta-lactam is not properly adjusted for a patient's renal function. Did you check your patient's renal function?
- All beta-lactams share a mechanism of action— inhibition of transpeptidases (i.e., penicillin-binding proteins) in the bacterial cell wall. Thus, giving two beta-lactams in combination for the same infection is generally not useful, but also not antagonistic (the penicillin-binding protein doesn't care which drug binds to it). There are a few exceptions to this rule, but not many.
- All beta-lactams lack activity against atypical organisms such as *Mycoplasma pneumoniae* and *Chlamydophila pneumoniae*. Add another drug to your regimen if you are concerned about these bugs, as in cases of community-acquired pneumonia.
- Nearly all currently available beta-lactams lack activity against MRSA. Add vancomycin or another agent if this bug is suspected (but note that its epidemiology is changing). Among

the available beta-lactams, only the cephalo-sporin ceftaroline has anti-MRSA activity. It is the exception that proves the rule.

Once you know the similarities among beta-lactams, it is easier to learn the differences among them.

Penicillins

Introduction to Penicillins

Penicillins are one of the largest and oldest classes of antimicrobial agents. Since the development of the natural penicillins in the 1930s, further penicillin development has been directed by the need to combat increasing antimicrobial resistance. Classes of penicillins with expanded Gram-negative spectra overcome the shortfalls of natural penicillins, and they can be grouped fairly easily by spectrum of activity.

Penicillins have several things in common:

- Penicillins have very short half-lives (< 2 hours) and must be dosed multiple times per day. The half-lives of most of them are prolonged in the presence of renal dysfunction.
- Like other beta-lactams, penicillins can cause hypersensitivity reactions. If a patient has a true IgE-mediated hypersensitivity reaction to a penicillin, other penicillins should be avoided, even if they are from different subclasses of penicillins. If the reaction is not severe, cephalosporins or carbapenems may be useful.
- Many penicillins are relatively poorly absorbed, even those available as oral formulations. This can lead to diarrhea when oral therapy

is needed. Pay attention to the dosing of oral versus intravenous (IV) penicillins—often, a conversion from IV to oral therapy means there will be a substantial decrease in the amount of active drug in the body.

Many penicillins were developed after the natural penicillins became available. Until researchers developed beta-lactamase inhibitors, development primarily focused on *either* improved activity against staphylococci (MSSA) or GNRs (Figure 7–1).

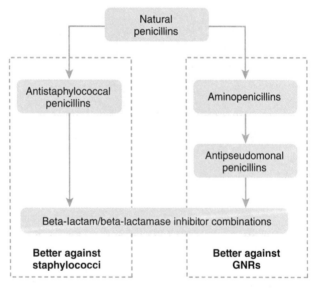

Figure 7–1
Penicillin Drug Development

Natural Penicillins

Agents: penicillin G, penicillin V

All of us have heard of the discovery of penicillin by Sir Alexander Fleming in 1929. Once penicillin was produced in medically useful quantities years later, it had a major impact on society, particularly in the treatment of wound infections. The importance of this discovery became apparent during World War II, when the Allies had access to life- and limb-saving penicillin and the Axis did not. Unfortunately, staphylococci quickly became resistant to penicillin through the production of penicillinases (beta-lactamases active against penicillins), initiating the search for new beta-lactams and leading to the confusing array of these drugs available today. The development of resistance has narrowed the spectrum of effectiveness of natural penicillins considerably over the past 60 years, such that staphylococci are almost universally resistant to them. Occasionally we still see an isolate of *Staphylococcus aureus* that does not produce penicillinase and is susceptible to penicillin.

Mechanism of Action

All beta-lactams inhibit cross-linking of peptidoglycan in the cell wall, leading to autolysis and cell death.

Spectrum

Good: Treponema pallidum, most streptococci, including *Streptococcus pneumoniae*

Moderate: enterococci

Poor: almost everything else

Adverse Effects

Similar to those of other beta-lactams.

Important Facts

- Natural penicillins have a very short half-life and must be dosed frequently or given by continuous infusion. Long-acting depot formulations (procaine, benzathine) are available for intramuscular administration. It is important to know the differences among these formulations because the doses vary considerably. It is even more important not to give procaine or benzathine products intravenously, which can be fatal.
- Penicillin V is the oral form of penicillin G. Other drugs have supplanted it in most uses, but not all.
- Penicillin G remains the drug of choice for syphilis.
- Because of resistance, penicillin is a poor empiric choice for most infections. Not all textbooks and references have been updated to reflect the changes in penicillin use that have resulted from widespread resistance.
- The intravenous penicillin breakpoint for *S. pneumoniae* were redefined in 2008 by CLSI (Clinical and Laboratory Standards Institute), which lowered the percentage of

S. pneumoniae isolates considered resistant to penicillin considerably. There are two caveats: (1) it only applies to intravenous penicillin and (2) it does not apply to central nervous system (CNS) infections, where the old breakpoints remain in effect. It is a practical reminder that breakpoints are useful predictors of treatment success, but they are not always set correctly.

What They're Good For

Syphilis, particularly neurosyphilis. During penicillin shortages, hospitals often reserve its use for this indication. Penicillin is also used in susceptible streptococcal infections such as pharyngitis or endocarditis.

Don't Forget!

Other, more conveniently dosed narrow-spectrum beta-lactams are available for most bugs treatable with penicillin.

Antistaphylococcal Penicillins

Agents: nafcillin, oxacillin, dicloxacillin, methicillin, cloxacillin

It did not take long for *Staphylococcus* species to become resistant to penicillin. Within a few years of penicillin becoming widely available, staphylococcal strains began to produce beta-lactamases, rendering penicillin useless in these infections. The basic structure of penicillin was modified to resist these destructive enzymes, leading to the antistaphylococcal penicillins. This modification gave these drugs activity against staphylococci that produce penicillinases, but did not add to the poor Gram-negative activity of the natural penicillins.

Mechanism of Action

All beta-lactams inhibit cross-linking of peptidoglycan in the cell wall, leading to autolysis and cell death.

Spectrum

Good: MSSA, streptococci
Poor: GNRs, enterococci, anaerobes, MRSA

Adverse Effects

Similar to those of other beta-lactams, with a possibly higher incidence of AIN.

Important Facts

- Antistaphylococcal penicillins have a short half-life and must be dosed frequently. This presents a problem, because they cause phlebitis. Does your patient have phlebitis? Try a first-generation cephalosporin instead. In general, they are easier to administer, better tolerated, and a good choice for most patients.
- Most antistaphylococcal penicillins are eliminated from the body in large part by the liver and do not need to be adjusted in cases of renal dysfunction.
- These drugs are interchangeable therapeutically. Therefore, *S. aureus* that is susceptible to methicillin (which is no longer used) is susceptible to oxacillin, nafcillin, and the rest. That is, MSSA = OSSA = NSSA, etc. Actually the "standard tests" are usually done with either oxacillin or cefoxitin.

What They're Good For

Infections caused by MSSA, such as endocarditis and skin and soft-tissue infections.

Don't Forget!

Beta-lactams kill staphylococci more quickly than vancomycin, so patients with MSSA infections who lack serious beta-lactam allergies should be switched to beta-lactams, such as antistaphylococcal penicillins or first-generation cephalosporins. This has been shown to be an important difference in serious infections.

Aminopenicillins

Agents: amoxicillin, ampicillin

Though the antistaphylococcal penicillins improve on the Gram-positive coverage of natural penicillins, they do not add to their Gram-negative coverage. Aminopenicillins are more water-soluble and pass through porin channels in the cell wall of some Gram-negative organisms. However, they are susceptible to beta-lactamases, and resistance to them has become fairly common in many regions of the world. Aminopenicillins are rarely active against staphylococci, because these almost always produce penicillinases. These drugs also do not have useful activity against *Pseudomonas aeruginosa*.

Mechanism of Action

All beta-lactams inhibit cross-linking of peptidoglycan in the cell wall, leading to autolysis and cell death.

Spectrum

Good: streptococci, enterococci
Moderate: enteric GNRs, *Haemophilus*
Poor: staphylococci, anaerobes, *Pseudomonas*

Adverse Effects

Similar to those of other beta-lactams. Aminopenicillins have a high incidence of diarrhea when given orally.

▓ Important Facts

- Though ampicillin can be given orally, amoxicillin is a better choice. It is more bioavailable, better tolerated, and administered less frequently. Use ampicillin for IV therapy and amoxicillin for oral therapy. Europeans disagree; they use amoxicillin intravenously also.
- Ampicillin is a drug of choice for susceptible enterococci. *Enterococcus faecalis* is almost always susceptible; *Enterococcus faecium* is often resistant.
- These drugs are often listed as alternative regimens for urinary tract infections (UTIs) in pregnant women because they are pregnancy category B and eliminated renally. However, resistance in *Escherichia coli* to them is very high and susceptibility testing should be performed. Always perform follow-up cultures in pregnant women with UTIs since even asymptomatic bacteruria is dangerous for them.

What They're Good For

Infections caused by susceptible GNRs, enterococci, and streptococci. Because resistance among GNRs is prevalent, aminopenicillins are used only infrequently in complicated nosocomial infections. Amoxicillin is frequently prescribed for infections of the upper respiratory tract, including streptococcal pharyngitis (strep throat) and otitis media (ear infection).

Don't Forget!

To achieve bactericidal activity against entero-cocci, ampicillin (or any other beta-lactam) has to be combined with an aminoglycoside. This should be done in serious infections such as endocarditis.

Antipseudomonal Penicillins

Agents: piperacillin, ticarcillin

None of the penicillins we have discussed thus far offer appreciable activity against *P. aeruginosa*, a common nosocomial pathogen that is often resistant to multiple antibiotics. Enter the antipseudomonal penicillins. These agents are active against *P. aeruginosa* and other more drug-resistant GNRs. However, they are just as susceptible to beta-lactamases as penicillin and ampicillin, so they are not antistaphylococcal. Also, strains of GNRs that produce beta-lactamases are resistant to them. They do have activity against streptococci and enterococci. They are now relevant only for a discussion of pharmacology, since they are rarely if ever used clinically by themselves.

Mechanism of Action

All beta-lactams inhibit cross-linking of peptidoglycan in the cell wall, leading to autolysis and cell death.

Spectrum

Good: *P. aeruginosa*, streptococci, enterococci
Moderate: enteric GNRs, *Haemophilus*
Poor: staphylococci, anaerobes

Adverse Effects

Similar to those of other beta-lactams.

Important Facts

- These drugs retain the Gram-positive activity of penicillin and are active against many streptococci and enterococci.
- None of the antipseudomonal penicillins are commonly used except in combination with a beta-lactamase inhibitor (see the next section).

What They're Good For

Taking up space in textbooks, since you won't find them on the pharmacy shelf.

Don't Forget!

When evaluating a penicillin/beta-lactamase inhibitor combination (see the next section), you need to understand the spectrum of the penicillin that the beta-lactamase inhibitor is protecting. That is why this section exists.

Penicillin/Beta-Lactamase Inhibitor Combinations

Agents: ampicillin/sulbactam, amoxicillin/clavulanate, piperacillin/tazobactam

Though the aminopenicillins and antipseudomonal penicillins have good intrinsic activity against GNRs, they remain just as susceptible to beta-lactamases as penicillin G. This means that they are not useful against the vast majority of staphylococci or many GNRs and anaerobes, because these organisms have learned to produce beta-lactamase. In other words, it seemed we learned either how to make a penicillin resistant to beta-lactamase, or how to make it more active against GNRs, but not both. Beta-lactamase inhibitors counter beta-lactamases; these drugs mimic the structure of beta-lactams but have little antimicrobial activity on their own. They bind to beta-lactamases irreversibly, preventing the beta-lactamase from destroying any beta-lactams that are coadministered and enabling the therapeutic beta-lactam to be effective.

When considering the activity of the beta-lactamase inhibitor combination, remember that the beta-lactamase inhibitor only frees up the beta-lactam to kill the organism—it doesn't enhance the activity. Therefore, the combination products are active only against the bacteria that the beta-lactam in the combination has intrinsic activity against. For example, ampicillin/sulbactam is active against beta-lactamase producing *E. coli*, because ampicillin alone is active against non-beta-lactamase producing *E. coli*. However, it has no useful activity against *Pseudomonas aeruginosa*, because ampicillin lacks activity against this organism. In contrast, piperacillin/tazobactam is active against *P. aeruginosa* because piperacillin alone is useful. Though these drugs have very broad spectra of activity, there are differences among the agents. Keep in mind the rule that beta-lactamase inhibitors restore activity, not add to it, to set them straight.

Mechanism of Action

All beta-lactams inhibit cross-linking of peptidoglycan in the cell wall, leading to autolysis and cell death. These beta-lactamase inhibitors structurally resemble beta-lactams and bind to many beta-lactamases, rendering them unable to inactivate the coadministered beta-lactam.

Spectrum

Good: MSSA, streptococci, enterococci, many anaerobes, enteric GNRs, *P. aeruginosa* (only piperacillin/tazobactam)

Moderate: GNRs with advanced beta-lactamases

Poor: MRSA, extended-spectrum beta-lactamase (ESBL) producing GNRs

Adverse Effects

Similar to those of other beta-lactams.

▨ Important Facts

- Unlike the other members of this class, amoxicillin/clavulanate is available orally. Various doses are available, but higher doses are associated with more diarrhea. Note that the dose of clavulanate is fixed in all oral dosage forms (125 mg).
- The beta-lactamase inhibitors packaged in these combinations are not active against all beta-lactamases. New beta-lactamases with the ability to destroy many types of beta-lactams are continually being discovered and are becoming more prevalent.
- Except for study purposes, beta-lactamase inhibitors are not available outside of the combination products.
- Sulbactam has useful activity against *Acinetobacter baumannii*, a highly drug-resistant GNR that causes nosocomial infections. For this reason, high doses of ampicillin/sulbactam can be used in the treatment of infections caused by this organism.
- Amoxicillin/clavulanate and ampicillin/sulbactam have nearly identical spectra of activity, but clavulanate is more potent at inhibiting beta-lactamases than sulbactam and higher doses of sulbactam are given to account for this fact. Differences in susceptibility testing may be due to the low concentrations of sulbactam used in tests.

What They're Good For

Empiric therapy of nosocomial infections, particularly nosocomial pneumonia (not aminopenicillin-based combinations). Because they have activity against aerobes and anaerobes, they are a good empiric choice for mixed infections, such as intra-abdominal infections, diabetic ulcers, and aspiration pneumonia. Amoxicillin/clavulanate is used for upper and lower respiratory tract infections when beta-lactamase–producing organisms are found or suspected. It can also be useful for UTIs when resistance to other drugs is seen, but it should not be given for a short 3-day course as with fluoroquinolones or TMP/SMX.

Don't Forget!

Narrow your coverage once culture results return. These are good choices of empiric therapy, but poor choices of definitive therapy if alternatives are available. Be sure you know which drugs are antipseudomonal and which are not—this is a major difference among these agents that drives their use. For example, ampicillin/sulbactam is a poor choice for nosocomial pneumonia, and piperacillin/tazobactam is overkill for community-acquired pneumonia.

Cephalosporins

Introduction to Cephalosporins

The cephalosporins are probably the most confusing group of antibiotics. For convenience, they have been grouped into "generations" that largely correlate with their spectrum of activity, with some notable exceptions. Although there are many different individual agents, the good news is that most hospitals use only a few of them, so, in practice, learning your institution's cephalosporin of choice is easy (outpatient pharmacies are a different story). In general, it is best to learn the characteristics of each generation and then learn the quirks about the individual agents. Figure 7–2 shows the general types of antimicrobial activity of the cephalosporin generations.

Cephalosporins have several elements in common:

* All are believed to have some cross-allergenicity with penicillins, though there are differences among generations. Estimates about the likelihood of cross-reactivity between penicillin and cephalosporin allergies differ. It is likely very low, below the oft-quoted 10%. A reasonable estimate is no more than 3–5%, though some publications support even lower

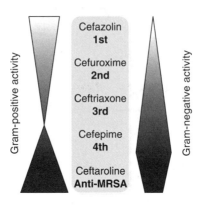

Figure 7–2
Cephalosporin Activity by Generation

numbers, particularly for later-generation agents. However, using any cephalosporin in a patient with a penicillin allergy is a matter of balancing risks and benefits. Assess the validity of the patient's allergy through interview and consider the level of risk associated with cephalosporin administration. Be skeptical of nausea, but be sure to take hives and any signs of anaphylaxis very seriously! Use alternative classes of antibiotics when practical. As mentioned earlier, evidence suggests that similar side chains are the reason for cross-reactivity, but this message isn't fully "out there" yet.

- The cephalosporins are generally more resistant to beta-lactamases than penicillins are. Beta-lactamases that are active against penicillins but inactive against cephalosporins are called *penicillinases*. Beta-lactamases that inactivate cephalosporins (*cephalosporinases*) also exist and are increasing in prevalence.

First-Generation Cephalosporins

First-generation cephalosporins are the most commonly used class of antibiotics in the hospital. Why? They are used immediately prior to surgery to prevent surgical site infections. Their spectrum of activity, inexpensive cost, and low incidence of adverse effects make them ideal for this purpose. For the same reasons, they are useful in treating skin and skin structure infections as well.

Mechanism of Action

All beta-lactams inhibit cross-linking of peptidoglycan in the cell wall, leading to autolysis and cell death.

Spectrum

Good: MSSA, streptococci
Moderate: some enteric GNRs
Poor: enterococci, anaerobes, MRSA, *Pseudomonas*

Adverse Effects

Similar to those of other beta-lactams.

Important Facts

- First-generation cephalosporins are good alternatives to antistaphylococcal penicillins. They cause less phlebitis and are infused less frequently. Unlike antistaphylococcal penicillins, however, they may not cross the blood–brain barrier and should not be used in CNS infections.
- Cephalexin and cefadroxil are available orally; the others are parenteral.

What They're Good For

Skin and skin structure infections, surgical prophylaxis, staphylococcal bloodstream infections, osteomyelitis, and endocarditis (MSSA).

Don't Forget!

Surgical prophylaxis is the most common indication for first-generation cephalosporins in the hospital. Be sure to limit the duration of therapy for this use; administering more than one dose of antibiotics should be the exception, and giving more than 24 hours of antibiotics is rarely justified. Such use does not lower infection rates, but it can select for more resistant organisms later in the hospital stay.

Second-Generation Cephalosporins

Agents: **cefuroxime, cefoxitin, cefotetan, cefprozil,** loracarbef, cefmetazole, cefonicid, cefamandole, cefaclor

Compared with first-generation cephalosporins, second-generation agents have better Gram-negative activity and somewhat weaker Gram-positive activity, though they are still used for these organisms. They are more stable against Gram-negative beta-lactamases and are particularly active against *Haemophilus influenzae* and *Neisseria gonorrhoeae*. Though the second-generation agents are the most numerous cephalosporins, they are probably the least utilized in practice in the United States.

Mechanism of Action

All beta-lactams inhibit cross-linking of peptidoglycan in the cell wall, leading to autolysis and cell death.

Spectrum

Good: some enteric GNRs, *Haemophilus, Neisseria*
Moderate: streptococci, staphylococci, anaerobes (only cefotetan, cefoxitin, cefmetazole)
Poor: enterococci, MRSA, *Pseudomonas*

Adverse Effects

Similar to those of other beta-lactams. Cephalosporins with the N-methylthiotetrazole (MTT) side chain—cefamandole, cefmetazole, and cefotetan—can inhibit vitamin K production and prolong bleeding. These MTT cephalosporins can also cause a disulfiram-like reaction when coadministered with ethanol. While *most* people in the hospital do not have access to alcoholic beverages while being treated for infections, outpatients need to be counseled on this interaction. It is a common question on board exams.

Important Facts

- Cefoxitin, cefotetan, and cefmetazole are cephamycins. They are grouped with the second-generation cephalosporins because they have similar activity, with one important exception: anaerobes. Cephamycins have activity against many anaerobes in the gastrointestinal (GI) tract, and cefoxitin and cefotetan are often used for surgical prophylaxis in abdominal surgery.
- Loracarbef is technically a carbacephem. You should immediately forget this to allow room for more important things.
- Cefaclor, cefprozil, and loracarbef are available only orally. Cefuroxime is available in both IV and oral formulations, and the others are IV only.
- Like first-generation cephalosporins, second-generation agents do not cross the blood–brain barrier well enough to be useful to treat CNS infections.

What They're Good For

Upper respiratory tract infections, community-acquired pneumonia, gonorrhea, surgical prophylaxis (cefotetan, cefoxitin, cefuroxime).

Don't Forget!

The cephamycins have good intrinsic anaerobic activity, but resistance to them is increasing in *Bacteroides fragilis* group infections. When using them for surgical prophylaxis, limit the duration of antibiotic exposure after surgery. If an infection does develop, use alternative agents such as beta-lactamase inhibitor combinations or another Gram-negative agent with metronidazole.

Third-Generation Cephalosporins

Agents: **ceftriaxone, cefotaxime, ceftazidime, cefdinir,** cefpodoxime, cefixime, ceftibuten

Third-generation cephalosporins have greater Gram-negative activity than the first- and second-generation drugs. Most of them also have good streptococcal activity, but generally lesser staphylococcal activity than previous generations of cephalosporins. These are broad-spectrum agents that have many different uses.

Mechanism of Action

All beta-lactams inhibit cross-linking of peptidoglycan in the cell wall, leading to autolysis and cell death.

Spectrum

Good: streptococci (except ceftazidime, which is poor), enteric GNRs, *Pseudomonas* (ceftazidime only)

Moderate: MSSA (except ceftazidime, which is poor)

Poor: enterococci, *Pseudomonas* (except ceftazidime), anaerobes, MRSA

Adverse Effects

Similar to those of other beta-lactams. Third-generation cephalosporins have been shown to be one of the classes of antibiotics with the strongest association with *Clostridium difficile*–associated diarrhea. Cefpodoxime has the MTT side chain that can inhibit vitamin K production (see section on second-generation cephalosporins for details).

Important Facts

- Ceftazidime is the exception to the spectrum of activity rule for third-generation agents. Unlike the others, it is antipseudomonal and lacks clinically useful activity against Gram-positive organisms.
- Ceftriaxone, cefotaxime, and ceftazidime cross the blood–brain barrier effectively and are useful for the treatment of CNS infections. However, their differences in activity lead clinicians to use them for different types of infections. Ceftazidime is a poor choice for community-acquired meningitis, in which *S. pneumoniae* predominates.
- Third-generation cephalosporins are notorious for inducing resistance among GNRs. Though they can be useful in nosocomial infections, too much broad-spectrum utilization can result in harder-to-treat organisms.
- A one-time dose of ceftriaxone 125 mg intramuscular (IM) has been a drug-of-choice for gonorrhea for many years, but the dose was increased to 250 mg IM due to increasing resistance. Patients treated for gonorrhea should receive azithromycin as well, which adds

empiric therapy for chlamydia and may reduce the emergence of ceftriaxone resistance.

- Ceftriaxone has the characteristic of having dual modes of elimination via both renal and biliary excretion. It does not need to be adjusted for renal dysfunction, but it does effectively treat UTIs.
- Ceftriaxone has two problems that make its use in neonates problematic: it interacts with calcium-containing medications to form crystals that can precipitate in the lungs and kidneys, which has led to fatalities, and it can also lead to biliary sludging with resultant hyperbilirubinemia. Avoid it—cefotaxime is a safer drug for these young patients.
- Last ceftriaxone fact: it should be given in higher doses of 2–4 g a day for MSSA infections, particularly invasive infections. Less activity against this organism means higher doses are recommended.

What They're Good For

Lower respiratory tract infections, pyelonephritis, nosocomial infections (ceftazidime), Lyme disease (ceftriaxone), meningitis, gonorrhea, skin and skin structure infections, febrile neutropenia (ceftazidime).

Don't Forget!

Ceftriaxone is a once-daily drug for almost all indications *except* meningitis. Make sure your meningitis patients receive the full 2 g IV q12h dose and also use vancomycin and ampicillin (if indicated). There are a few more indications for the high dose, but meningitis is the most important one.

Fourth-Generation Cephalosporins

Agent: cefepime

There is only one fourth-generation cephalosporin, cefepime. Cefepime is the broadest-spectrum cephalosporin, with activity against both Gram-negative organisms, including *Pseudomonas*, and Gram-positive organisms. One way to remember its spectrum is to think that cefazolin (1st) + ceftazidime (3rd) = cefepime (4th).

Mechanism of Action

All beta-lactams inhibit cross-linking of peptidoglycan in the cell wall, leading to autolysis and cell death.

Spectrum

Good: MSSA, streptococci, *Pseudomonas*, enteric GNRs
Moderate: Acinetobacter
Poor: enterococci, anaerobes, MRSA

Adverse Effects

Generally, similar to those of other beta-lactams, but cefepime may be associated with more neurotoxicity than other agents.

Important Facts

- Cefepime is a broad-spectrum agent. It is a good empiric choice for many nosocomial infections, but it is overkill for most community-acquired infections. Be sure to deescalate therapy if possible when you treat empirically with cefepime.
- For monotherapy of febrile neutropenia, cefepime is a better choice than ceftazidime because of its better Gram-positive activity. It may also induce less resistance in GNRs than third-generation cephalosporins, but it is still not a good drug to overuse.
- Cefepime briefly had a bad reputation after a meta-analysis showed increased mortality with its use compared with other drugs. Many clinicians were skeptical, however, and a more thorough FDA analysis exonerated cefepime.
- Neurotoxicity with cefepime can occur and may manifest as nonconvulsive status epilepticus. It can occur at any dose, but dose adjustment of the drug for patients with renal dysfunction is important.

What It's Good For

Febrile neutropenia, nosocomial pneumonia, postneurosurgical meningitis, other nosocomial infections.

Don't Forget!

Cefepime is used primarily for nosocomial infections. Although it is indicated for infections of the urinary tract and lower respiratory tract, it is overkill for most community-acquired sources of these infections.

Anti-MRSA Cephalosporins

Ceftaroline is a cephalosporin that has unique characteristics that defy the "generational" label. The CLSI has designated it an "anti-MRSA cephalosporin," which we're going with since it highlights the most important characteristic of the drug. What makes this agent unique is activity against MRSA. Its structure has been engineered to bind to the penicillin-binding protein 2a of MRSA that has low affinity for other beta-lactams. Unlike other cephalosporins, ceftaroline also has modest activity against *E. faecalis* (but not *E. faecium*). It lost some of the Gram-negative potency of cefepime and has Gram-negative activity similar to that of ceftriaxone. In an era of high MRSA prevalence, ceftaroline offers an intriguing possibility for therapy, but because it is fairly new its role is not yet defined. Another agent with similar characteristics exists (ceftobiprole), but it was removed from the market in the few countries in which it was approved after U.S. and E.U. regulators did not approve it.

Mechanism of Action

All beta-lactams inhibit cross-linking of peptidoglycan in the cell wall, leading to autolysis and cell death. Unlike other beta-lactams, ceftaroline can bind to penicillin-binding protein 2a, a type that is expressed by MRSA. This characteristic is responsible for its anti-MRSA activity.

Spectrum

Good: MSSA, MRSA, streptococci, enteric GNRs
Moderate: E. faecalis
Poor: P. aeruginosa, E. faecium, Acinetobacter, anaerobes

Adverse Effects

Information available to date from clinical trials suggests adverse effects of ceftaroline are similar to those of other beta-lactams.

Important Facts

- As is typical for new antimicrobials coming to market, the initial indications for ceftaroline are "low-hanging fruit": skin and skin structure infections and community-acquired pneumonia. These are indications for which there are already a great many agents available, though ceftaroline outperformed ceftriaxone in community-acquired pneumonia in two of the three studies. The challenge will be to determine what the role of ceftaroline is for hospital-acquired pneumonia and other severe diseases often caused by drug-resistant pathogens. Ceftaroline has been described in case series and retrospective studies to successfully treat bloodstream infections, endocarditis, meningitis, osteomyelitis, and hospital-acquired pneumonia.

What it's Good For

Ceftaroline is approved (in the United States) for treatment of complicated skin and soft tissue infections and community-acquired pneumonia. There are less rigorous data for other uses.

Don't Forget!

Some references are describing ceftaroline as a fifth-generation cephalosporin (including us just one edition ago). If you choose to categorize it this way, just don't forget that its Gram-negative activity is less compared to the fourth generation, especially as regards *P. aeruginosa*.

Cephalosporin/Beta-Lactamase Inhibitor Combinations

Agents: ceftazidime/avibactam, ceftolozane/tazobactam

Carbapenems, the subject of the next section, have been drugs of choice for some of our most resistant GNRs for many years, so it was no surprise when resistance to them began to emerge. Carbapenem resistance is mostly seen in three key organisms that commonly cause infection: *Klebsiella pneumoniae, P. aeruginosa,* and *A. baumannii.* Avibactam is a new type of beta-lactamase inhibitor with a mechanism of action that is different from other beta-lactamase inhibitors and that works against many beta-lactamases produced by *K. pneumoniae* and *P. aeruginosa.* It restores the activity of ceftazidime against many of these organisms. Ceftolozane is a third-generation cephalosporin that evades many resistance mechanisms of *P. aeruginosa*, and tazobactam is given with it to protect it from some beta-lactamases. Neither of the agents have good activity against *Acinetobacter*. Note the differences in the spectrum of these agents since they dictate their uses in different situations.

Mechanism of Action

All beta-lactams inhibit cross-linking of peptido-glycan in the cell wall, leading to autolysis and cell death. Tazobactam is a beta-lactamase inhibitor that structurally resembles beta-lactams and binds to many beta-lactamases, rendering them unable to inactivate the coadministered beta-lactam. Avibactam does not resemble a beta-lactam, but it also binds beta-lactamases and renders them inert.

Spectrum

Good: Pseudomonas, enteric GNRs (ceftazidime/avibactam > ceftolozane/tazobactam)

Moderate: some streptococci (ceftolozane/tazobactam)

Poor: most anaerobes, MRSA, MSSA, *Acinetobacter*

Adverse Effects

Similar to those of other beta-lactams.

▓ Important Facts

- There are minor, but important differences in the spectrum of activity between these two drugs. Both are active against most multidrug-resistant *Pseudomonas*, but only ceftazidime/avibactam is active against carbapenem-resistant *Klebsiella* and other enteric GNRs. This difference dictates how they are used in clinical practice.
- Both agents evade many mechanisms of resistance of *Pseudomonas*, but in different ways. Ceftolozane itself is minimally affected by many *Pseudomonas*-resistance mechanisms, including its beta-lactamase—tazobactam itself adds

little for this bug. Ceftazidime/avibactam relies on avibactam to inactivate beta-lactamases produced by *Pseudomonas*. It is possible to see isolates of *Pseudomonas* that are resistant to one of these drugs and susceptible to the other.

- Unlike penicillin-based beta-lactamase inhibitor combinations like piperacillin/tazobactam, there is substantial resistance to these agents among gut anaerobes. If you suspect anaerobic involvement in your patient and you are using one of these agents, add metronidazole.

What They're Good For

- *Both:* multidrug-resistant *Pseudomonas* infections, mixed aerobic/anaerobic infections, infections caused by ESBL-producing organisms, intra-abdominal infections
- *Ceftazidime / avibactam:* carbapenem-resistant Enterobacteriaceae infections

Don't Forget!

Even though these are new drugs and highly active against resistant GNRs, resistance to them does occur. Ask your lab to test them for your patient's isolate. The bugs never give up.

Carbapenems

Agents: imipenem/cilastatin, meropenem, ertapenem, doripenem

Carbapenems are our broadest-spectrum antibacterial drugs, particularly imipenem, doripenem, and meropenem. They possess a beta-lactam ring and share the same mechanism of action of beta-lactams, but they are structurally unique and differ from both penicillins and cephalosporins. Their broad spectrum makes them both appealing and unappealing for empiric therapy, depending on the infection being treated and the risk factors of the patient for a resistant organism. Imipenem, doripenem, and meropenem have similar spectra of activity; ertapenem has important differences in its spectrum that must be learned.

Mechanism of Action

All beta-lactams inhibit cross-linking of peptidoglycan in the cell wall, leading to autolysis and cell death.

Spectrum

Good: MSSA, streptococci, anaerobes, enteric GNRs, *Pseudomonas* (not ertapenem), *Acinetobacter* (not ertapenem), ESBL-producing GNRs

Moderate: enterococci (not ertapenem)
Poor: MRSA, penicillin-resistant streptococci

Adverse Effects

Similar to those of other beta-lactams, but imipenem has a higher propensity to induce seizures. Minimize the risk by calculating appropriate doses for patients with renal dysfunction and avoiding imipenem use in patients with meningitis, because it can cross the blood–brain barrier more readily.

Important Facts

- Imipenem is metabolized in the kidney to a nephrotoxic product. Cilastatin blocks the renal dehydropeptidase that catalyzes this reaction and prevents this metabolism from occurring. It is always coadministered with imipenem for this reason.
- Carbapenems are very broad-spectrum agents. Imipenem, doripenem, and meropenem are particularly broad and should not be used empirically for most community-acquired infections. They are good choices for many types of nosocomial infections, particularly in patients who have received many other classes of antibiotics during their hospital stay.
- Although ertapenem has weaker activity than the other carbapenems for a few organisms, this activity is significant enough to change the utility of the drug (think: **E**rtapenem is the **E**xception). Ertapenem is a poor choice for many nosocomial infections, particularly nosocomial pneumonia in which both *Pseudomonas*

and *Acinetobacter* are important pathogens. However, it is administered only once a day and thus more convenient than the other carbapenems, so it may be a better choice for home-infusion therapy for susceptible infections.

- Carbapenems may uncommonly elicit an allergic reaction in patients with a history of penicillin allergy. One study showed the incidence of such reactions to be as high as 47% with a proven penicillin allergy (keep in mind that many penicillin allergies are unproven), but more recent and better-performed studies in patients with anaphylaxis to penicillin have shown this number to be *much* lower (close to 1%). However, keep in mind that even if the cross-reactivity is very low between these agents, patients with a history of allergy to *any* drug are more likely to react to another one even if they are not related.
- Carbapenemases that render these drugs inert exist and are becoming more common. In the United States they are most common in the Northeast; they are very common in some other parts of the world. Both imipenem/cilastatin and meropenem are being studied in combination with new beta-lactamase inhibitors that restore their activity against carbapenemase-producing GNRs.

What They're Good For

All: mixed aerobic/anaerobic infections, infections caused by ESBL-producing organisms, intra-abdominal infections

Imipenem, doripenem, meropenem: nosocomial pneumonia, febrile neutropenia, other nosocomial infections

Don't Forget!

Check your dosing in patients with renal dysfunction to minimize the risk of imipenem-induced seizures.

Monobactams

aztreonam

Aztreonam is the only monobactam currently available. Structurally, aztreonam contains only the four-membered ring of the basic beta-lactam structure, hence the name monobactam. Aztreonam's quirk is that it seems to be safe to administer to patients with allergies to other beta-lactams, except patients who have a specific allergy to ceftazidime. This cross-reactivity seems to be a result of the fact that ceftazidime and aztreonam share an identical side chain (note: ceftolozane also shares this side chain). Ceftazidime and aztreonam also share virtually the same spectrum of activity. It is reasonably safe to remember the utility of aztreonam by thinking of it as ceftazidime without allergic cross-reactivity with other beta-lactams.

Mechanism of Action

Like the other beta-lactams, monobactams inhibit cross-linking of peptidoglycan in the cell wall, leading to autolysis and cell death.

Spectrum

Good: Pseudomonas, most GNRs
Moderate: Acinetobacter
Poor: Gram-positive organisms, anaerobes

Adverse Effects

Similar to those of other beta-lactams, but with a low incidence of hypersensitivity.

Important Facts

- Aztreonam shares a mechanism of action and pharmacodynamic profile with other beta-lactams. Because it is a Gram-negative drug that is often used in patients with penicillin allergies, it is often confused with aminoglycosides. It is chemically unrelated to aminoglycosides and does not share their toxicities.
- Aztreonam can be administered via inhalation to patients with cystic fibrosis to prevent exacerbations of infection.
- Aztreonam is a type of beta-lactam, and combination therapy with it and other beta-lactams against the same organism is unwarranted. Try adding a non-beta-lactam drug to your empiric regimen for serious nosocomial infections instead.

What It's Good For

Gram-negative infections, including *Pseudomonas*, particularly in patients with a history of beta-lactam allergy.

Don't Forget!

Before using aztreonam in your patients with beta-lactam allergies, investigate whether the reaction was specifically to ceftazidime. If you cannot determine this and the reaction was serious, proceed with caution or use an alternative agent.

Glycopeptides and Short-Acting Lipoglycopeptides

8

Agents: vancomycin, telavancin

To date, three glycopeptides are in clinical use: vancomycin, teicoplanin, and telavancin. Teicoplanin is not available in the United States, and telavancin was recently approved.

Vancomycin is invaluable, because it has activity against most things Gram-positive that have not learned to become resistant to it. Many enterococci (especially *Enterococcus faecium*) have figured this out—we call them vancomycin-resistant enterococci (VRE). A few staphylococci have learned vancomycin resistance from the enterococci, but these staphylococci are currently very rare. In general, they are susceptible.

Telavancin is a somewhat different agent. It is a lipoglycopeptide that was modified from vancomycin's structure. It has some unique properties that may be advantageous compared with vancomycin, such as improved activity against MRSA that is less susceptible to vancomycin, but its place in therapy is still being determined.

Mechanism of Action

Glycopeptides bind to terminal D-ala-D-ala chains on peptidoglycan in the cell well, preventing further elongation of peptidoglycan chains. Telavancin has a second mechanism where the drug interferes with the cell membrane also, disrupting membrane function.

Spectrum

Good: MSSA, MRSA, streptococci, *Clostridium difficile*
Moderate: enterococci
Poor: anything Gram-negative

Adverse Effects

Infusion-related reactions: A histamine-mediated reaction called red man syndrome is classically associated with vancomycin. When it occurs, the patient may feel warm, flushed, and may develop hypotension. This reaction can be prevented by slowing the infusion rate and is not a true allergy. Antihistamines can also ameliorate the reaction. Because the core structure of telavancin is essentially vancomycin, it may cause this reaction as well.

Ototoxicity: Vancomycin has historically been considered an ototoxic drug, but evidence linking it with this toxicity is unclear.

Renal: Nephrotoxicity is an adverse effect classically assigned to vancomycin. Although the historical evidence linking this with vancomycin is poor, recent studies have shown that it may be nephrotoxic in higher doses, including the higher doses that are commonly used to treat MRSA infections in the twenty-first century. The early formulation of vancomycin was brown, and clinicians trying to amuse themselves dubbed it "Mississippi mud." The current formulation is clear and lacks those potentially toxic excipients. Telavancin has renal toxicity issues as well.

Telavancin: In addition to the above reactions, taste disturbances and foamy urine occur with telavancin. Telavancin should not be given to pregnant women because of problems seen in animal studies.

Dosing Issues

Vancomycin is often pharmacokinetically monitored. Trough concentrations are often used to ensure that the drug is not being eliminated too quickly or slowly, and different indications have different preferred trough ranges. Recent data indicate that higher troughs may be associated with nephrotoxicity. Peak concentrations are only useful for calculating patient-specific pharmacokinetic parameters. They do not seem to predict efficacy or safety and should not be drawn for most patients.

Important Facts

- Oral vancomycin is absorbed very poorly. Its only use is for the treatment of *Clostridium difficile*–associated disease. Also, IV vancomycin does not reach intracolonic concentrations high enough to kill *C. difficile*, so oral is the only way to go.
- Oral vancomycin achieves gut concentrations that are sky-high, so the lowest dose is the best one for the majority of patients.
- Do not overreact if your vancomycin trough is too high. Was it drawn correctly? If so, increase your dosing interval.
- Although vancomycin is active against staphylococci, it does not kill MSSA as quickly

as beta-lactams do. Does your patient have MSSA? Use cefazolin or nafcillin instead.

- Recently, a phenomenon described as "MIC creep" has been seen with staphylococci and vancomycin. MICs have been rising to vancomycin in many institutions, and while they have not yet reached the level of resistance, they are increasing within the range labeled as susceptible, that is, ≤ 2 mg/L. However, some data shows that patients receiving vancomycin for serious infections caused by staphylococci with an MIC = 2 mg/L to vancomycin have worse outcomes than those with lower MICs. This issue warrants careful attention.

- Telavancin is more rapidly bactericidal than vancomycin. This activity may be an advantage in the treatment of some infections, but clinical evidence that shows a benefit is lacking at this point. It may be useful for patients not responding to other therapies for MRSA infections.

- Even though it is pregnancy category C, telavancin should not be used in pregnant women unless absolutely necessary since developmental issues were seen in animals.

What They're Good For

Vancomycin is a drug of choice for MRSA infections and for empiric use when MRSA is a concern, such as for nosocomial pneumonia. It is also useful in other Gram-positive infections when the patient has a severe beta-lactam allergy. Telavancin is indicated for skin and skin structure infections and hospital-acquired pneumonia. Its role is still being defined.

Don't Forget!

Are you *sure* that vancomycin trough concentration was drawn correctly? Mistimed vancomycin levels are very common!

Long-Acting Glycopeptides

9

Agents: dalbavancin, oritavancin

Dalbavancin and oritavancin are unique agent. Pharmacologically, they start with the base structure of a glycopeptide and have been designed with pharmacokinetic characteristics that slow their elimination. Both can be dosed intravenously just once for the equivalent of 2 weeks of therapy since each has a half-life of over a week.

Both drugs have strictly Gram-positive activity that includes MRSA and streptococci. This begs the question of where one would use drugs like these? Right now, they are both indicated for infections of the skin and skin structure, where both *Staphylococcus* and *Streptococcus* cause most infections. There is a lot of appeal to giving patients just one dose of drug for a full course of therapy (think about compliance!), but it comes with a price. They are cheaper than a hospital admission, but the cost of a single dose could buy you a Hawaiian vacation!

Mechanism of Action

All glycopeptides bind to terminal D-ala-D-ala chains on peptidoglycan in the cell well, preventing further elongation of peptidoglycan chains. Lipoglycopeptides have a second mechanism where the drug interferes with the cell membrane also, disrupting membrane function.

Spectrum

Good: MSSA, MRSA, streptococci, enterococci (oritavancin)

Moderate: enterococci (dalbavancin)

Poor: anything Gram-negative

Adverse Effects

In clinical trials, nausea, vomiting, diarrhea, and rash were the most common adverse effects with both drugs. Infusion-related reactions can occur with oritavancin if it is infused quickly, so it is given over 3 hours.

Oritavancin inhibits warfarin metabolism and may increase the risk of bleeding when given with it.

Important Facts

- The prolonged elimination of these drugs is a significant advantage that can enable easy outpatient options and ensure "compliance" (by forcing it upon the patient with the infusion). However, these patients still need to be monitored for both treatment success and adverse effects.

- Oritavancin interferes with assays for prothrombin time (PT) for 24 hours and activated partial thromboplastin time (aPTT) for 48 hours, which are used to monitor warfarin and heparin, respectively. These drugs should not be used in combination with oritavancin during those time periods since monitoring will be unreliable.

- Dalbavancin has different dosing depending on if it is administered twice (1000 mg on day 1, then 500 mg a week later) or once (1500 mg). Why would one use the two-dose regimen, you ask? We don't know, but it was studied first.

What They're Good For

Skin and skin structure infections in patients whose infections are either known or highly suspected to be caused by Gram-positive organisms. The paradigm for which patients are best for these interesting drugs is still being defined.

Don't Forget!

Patients discharged on these drugs still need monitoring—it's not just "set it and... forget it!"

Fluoroquinolones

10

From a spectrum of activity and pharmacokinetic standpoint, many of the fluoroquinolones are near-ideal antibiotics: they have broad-spectrum activity that includes Gram-positive, Gram-negative, and atypical organisms; display excellent oral bioavailability; and distribute widely into tissues. Unfortunately, these characteristics have led to overprescribing and the inevitable rise in resistance, despite recommendations to reserve this class. In particular, although activity against enteric Gram-negative organisms (such as *Escherichia coli* and *Klebsiella*) historically has been excellent, in some geographical regions and patient populations these drugs have lost much of their activity, and they are no longer recommended in the United States as first-line drugs for uncomplicated urinary tract infections (UTIs). The newer drugs (moxifloxacin, gemifloxacin) gain increasing Gram-positive (mostly pneumococcal) activity at the expense of some Gram-negative (mostly *Pseudomonas*) activity. Significant differences among the agents are in **bold**.

Mechanism of Action

Fluoroquinolones inhibit DNA topoisomerases, enzymes that are involved in winding and unwinding the DNA; the action of the fluoroquinolones can lead to breaks in the DNA and death of the cell.

Spectrum: ciprofloxacin

Good: enteric GNRs (*E. coli, Proteus, Klebsiella,* etc.), *Haemophilus influenzae*

Moderate: Pseudomonas, atypicals (*Mycoplasma, Chlamydia, Legionella*)

Poor: staphylococci, *Streptococcus pneumoniae*, anaerobes, enterococci

Spectrum: levofloxacin/moxifloxacin/ gemifloxacin

Good: enteric Gram negatives, **S. pneumoniae,** atypicals, *H. influenzae*

Moderate: Pseudomonas (**levofloxacin only**), MSSA

Poor: anaerobes (**except moxifloxacin**, which has moderate activity), enterococci

Adverse Effects

Nervous system: Fluoroquinolones can cause central nervous system (CNS) adverse reactions, including dizziness, confusion, and hallucinations. Elderly patients are particularly susceptible to these. Younger patients may develop insomnia. Peripheral neuropathy can also occur.

Cardiovascular: Prolongation of the QT interval can be observed, but arrhythmias usually only occur in patients with other risk factors (underlying arrhythmia, concomitant proar-rhythmic drug, excessive dose).

Musculoskeletal: Arthralgias (uncommonly) and Achilles tendon rupture (very rarely) may occur. Tendon rupture is more common in the elderly, patients with renal dysfunction, and those taking corticosteroids. Tendonitis usu-ally precedes rupture, so complaints of tendon pain should be taken seriously. Less commonly, exacerbations of myasthenia gravis may occur.

Dermatologic: Photosensitivity is often seen. Patients should avoid the sun or use sunscreen while taking fluoroquinolones.

Developmental: Because of toxicities seen in juve-nile beagle dogs, fluoroquinolones are contra-indicated in pregnant women and relatively contraindicated in children, although experience with use in children suggests they may be used.

Important Facts

- While ciprofloxacin and levofloxacin have activ-ity against *Pseudomonas*, MICs are typically higher than with other susceptible organisms (e.g., *E. coli*). Thus, when using these drugs to treat documented or possible *Pseudomonas* infections, give them at higher, antipseudomonal doses: 400 mg IV q8h or 750 mg PO q12h for ciprofloxacin; 750 mg IV/PO daily for levofloxacin.
- Bioavailability of all fluoroquinolones is 80–100%, so oral dose = IV dose (**except ciprofloxacin**: PO = ~1.25 times IV dose).
- Levofloxacin and ciprofloxacin are the *only* drugs that are well-absorbed and active against *Pseudomonas*, but resistance to them

is unfortunately common for this pathogen. Susceptibility testing is a must.

- Fluoroquinolones chelate cations, and their oral bioavailability is *significantly decreased* when administered with calcium, iron, antacids, milk, or multivitamins. Separate these agents by at least 2 hours or have your patient take a week off of the supplements, if possible. Administration with tube feedings is also problematic. This problem is unique to the oral formulations—IV forms avoid it.

- Most fluoroquinolones are cleared renally and require dose reduction in renal dysfunction. **Moxifloxacin is the exception**; because it is not excreted into the urine, it is also not approved for treatment of UTIs. Gemifloxacin has dual elimination, and its utility in treating UTIs is not established, though it does require dose adjustment in renal failure. It is probably best to avoid using gemifloxacin for UTIs until there is evidence that supports its use.

- The FDA mandates a boxed warning to all fluoroquinolone package inserts regarding the possibility of tendon rupture.

- Important note: in 2016, FDA required the addition of a warning for all systemic fluoroquinolones that their risks outweigh their benefits for most cases of sinusitis, bronchitis, and uncomplicated UTIs unless other options are not available. This is due to the possibility of rare but serious adverse effects, including those listed above.

What They're Good For

Not everything, despite the temptation. Remember, the longer you want to be able to use these drugs, the more restraint should be exercised now. Indications for the fluoroquinolones are listed in Table 10–1.

Don't Forget!

When using the oral forms of fluoroquinolones, be especially careful to avoid coadministering with chelating agents (calcium, magnesium, aluminum, etc.).

TABLE 10–1
Indications for Fluoroquinolones

Indication	Cipro	Levo	Moxi	Gemi
CAP, sinusitis, AECB	−	+	+	+
UTI	+	+	−	?
Intra-abdominal infection	+	+	+	?
Systemic Gram-negative infections	+	+	+	?
Skin/soft tissue infection	−	+	+	+
Pseudomonas infections (+/− beta-lactam)	+	+	−	−
Treatment/prophylaxis in bioterrorism scenarios (active vs. anthrax, plague, tularemia)	+	+	?	?

+ = approved/studied/makes sense for this indication.
? = should work, no clinical data.
− = suboptimal.

11

Aminoglycosides

Agents: gentamicin, tobramycin, amikacin, streptomycin, spectinomycin

The aminoglycosides as a class dispel the notion that antibiotics are largely nontoxic. These drugs have a narrow therapeutic window, and improper dosing carries the risk of inflicting significant toxicity (primarily nephro- and ototoxicity) on your patients. Because of this, there has been a reduction in their use as primary therapy for most infections. That being said, they retain good activity against many problem pathogens (such as *Pseudomonas* and *Acinetobacter*) that have developed resistance to the more benign drug classes. They are also excellent at synergizing with the beta-lactams and glycopeptides to improve the efficiency of bacterial killing. Gentamicin and tobramycin are the most widely used drugs, amikacin is generally reserved for pathogens resistant to the first two, and streptomycin has limited uses (*Enterococcus*, tuberculosis, and plague).

Mechanism of Action

Aminoglycosides bind to the bacterial ribosome (the 30S subunit, if you must know), causing misreading of the genetic code, leading to incorrect protein formation and interruption of protein synthesis.

Spectrum: gentamicin/tobramycin/amikacin

Good: Gram-negatives (*Escherichia coli, Klebsiella, Pseudomonas, Acinetobacter*, most others)

Moderate: in combination with a beta-lactam or glycopeptide: staphylococci (including MRSA), viridans streptococci, enterococci (gentamicin and streptomycin are best)

Poor: atypicals, anaerobes, Gram-positive organisms (as monotherapy)

Adverse Effects

Nephrotoxicity: Oliguric acute renal failure, preceded by a rising serum creatinine, is a dose-related adverse effect of aminoglycosides. Risk can be reduced by correct dosing (including the use of extended-interval dosing), as well as avoidance of coadministration of other nephrotoxins (cyclosporine, cisplatin, foscarnet, etc.).

Ototoxicity: Aminoglycosides cause dose-related cochlear and vestibular toxicity. For patients anticipated to receive long-term ($\geq$ 2 weeks) of aminoglycosides, baseline and follow-up audiology are necessary. It is important to monitor patients closely for any hearing loss or balance problems, because these are not reversible and can significantly affect quality of life.

Neurologic: Neuromuscular blockade can occur when aminoglycosides are given, particularly in high doses to patients who are receiving therapeutic paralysis.

▪ Important Facts

- Once-daily or extended-interval aminoglycoside dosing leverages the concentration-dependent killing of the drugs to create an equally effective, more convenient, and possibly safer dosing regimen. However, there are many populations in which once-daily dosing has had less study, including the pregnant, the critically ill, those with significant renal dysfunction, and the morbidly obese. Use this dosing method with caution, if at all, in these populations. Aminoglycosides are pregnancy category D and should be avoided if possible in pregnant women anyway.

- Aminoglycoside serum levels can help guide appropriate dosing and reduce the risk of toxicity, but they must be drawn correctly to have meaningful interpretations. For traditional dosing methods, a peak level should be drawn half an hour after the end of the infusion, while trough levels should be drawn within 30 minutes of the next dose. For once-daily dosing there are a number of potential monitoring points, based on published nomograms.

- Aminoglycosides have relatively poor distribution to many tissues, including the lungs and central nervous system. This makes them less than optimal as monotherapy for many severe infections. It also means that a dose should be based on the patient's ideal or adjusted body weight, rather than his or her total body weight. Given the high prevalence of morbid obesity, serious overdosing of patients can occur if the patient's total body weight is used.

- There are minor differences between the aminoglycosides in their activity:
  - For *Pseudomonas*: amikacin> tobramycin > gentamicin.
  - For *Klebsiella*: amikacin = gentamicin > tobramycin.

- Some older drug references and textbooks list streptomycin as a first-line treatment for tuberculosis. While it was the first antituberculosis drug available, it has been supplanted by safer and more effective first-line drugs. It is still an alternative in resistant tuberculosis infections—these should be treated by an expert in their management.

What They're Good For

In combination with a beta-lactam agent, treatment of serious infections with documented or suspected Gram-negative pathogens, including febrile neutropenia, sepsis, exacerbations of cystic fibrosis, and ventilator-associated pneumonia. Aminoglycosides, primarily gentamicin, are also used in combination with a beta-lactam or glycopeptide for treatment of serious Gram-positive infections, including endocarditis, osteomyelitis, and sepsis. In combination with other antimycobacterials, they are used for treatment of drug-resistant infections with *Mycobacterium tuberculosis* or other mycobacteria (streptomycin and amikacin).

Don't Forget!

Most aminoglycoside toxicity is dose related, so get the dose right from the start by adjusting for renal dysfunction and using ideal or adjusted body weight. Pharmacokinetic concentrations are useful for monitoring and dosing aminoglycosides if they are drawn correctly.

Tetracyclines and Glycylcyclines

12

Once considered broad-spectrum antibiotics, the relentless advance of bacterial resistance and the off-patent status of the drugs have reduced the use of tetracyclines to niche indications. They are useful (but not highly studied) alternatives for the treatment of common respiratory tract infections and drugs of choice for a variety of uncommon infections. Doxycycline is preferred in most situations over tetracycline and minocycline. The glycylcyclines (tigecycline being the first agent in the class) evade most tetracycline resistance mechanisms and have a broad spectrum of activity.

Mechanism of Action

Tetracyclines and glycyclines both bind to the bacterial ribosome at the 30S subunit, preventing the docking of transfer RNA carrying new amino acids for addition to the elongating protein chain.

Spectrum: tetracycline/doxycycline/minocycline

Good: atypicals, rickettsia, spirochetes (e.g., *Borrelia burgdorferi, Helicobacter pylori*), *Plasmodium* species (malaria)

Moderate: staphylococci (including MRSA), *Streptococcus pneumoniae*

Poor: most GNRs, anaerobes, enterococci

Spectrum: tigecycline

Good: atypicals, enterococci (including VRE), staphylococci (including MRSA), *S. pneumoniae*

Acceptable: most GNRs, anaerobes

Poor: Pseudomonas, Proteus, Providencia (see a **p-p-p**attern?)

Adverse Effects

Gastrointestinal: Tetracyclines can cause esophageal irritation, and patients should take the drug with water, while standing up if possible. Tigecycline, though an IV drug, can cause severe nausea, vomiting, and diarrhea.

Dermatologic: Photosensitivity is often seen. Patients should avoid the sun or use sunscreen while taking tetracyclines.

Sensory: Minocycline may cause dizziness and vertigo.

Developmental: All tetracyclines can cause discoloration of developing teeth and are contraindicated in pregnant women and children younger than 8 years old.

Important Facts

- Doxycycline and minocycline bioavailability is approximately 100%. Tigecycline is IV only.
- Tetracyclines chelate cations, and their oral bioavailability is *decreased significantly* when administered with calcium, iron, antacids, or

multivitamins. Have patients separate these agents by at least 2 hours or take a week off from the supplements, if possible. Food decreases the absorption of tetracycline substantially, but of minocycline and doxycycline minimally.

- Doxycycline does not need to be adjusted in renal or hepatic dysfunction; tetracycline is eliminated renally and should not be used in cases of renal insufficiency (it can worsen renal dysfunction).
- Tigecycline has a very large volume of distribution, indicating that it distributes highly into many tissues. However, it is eliminated hepatically, achieves low urinary concentrations, and probably should not be used for UTIs. Its extensive distribution also leads to low bloodstream concentrations, and it is not an ideal choice for treating primary bloodstream infections.
- An analysis performed by the FDA across all indications for tigecycline showed it to have a mortality disadvantage compared to the other antibiotics studied. This was driven largely by a study of hospital-acquired pneumonia. While this is obviously concerning, tigecycline still may be useful because it has activity against many highly drug-resistant organisms in which there are few (or no) alternatives. Those types of infections usually do not make it into clinical studies.

What They're Good For

Uncomplicated respiratory tract infections: acute exacerbations of chronic bronchitis, sinusitis, and community-acquired pneumonia. They are drugs of choice for many tick-borne diseases. Use as alternative drugs for skin or soft-tissue infections, syphilis, pelvic inflammatory disease (with cefoxitin). Use as an alternative to ciprofloxacin in bioterrorism scenarios (they are active against anthrax, plague, and tularemia). Use for malaria prophylaxis and treatment. Tigecycline may have a role in the treatment of complicated polymicrobial infections, such as intra-abdominal infections and complicated skin and skin structure infections.

Don't Forget!

Ask patients if they take mineral supplements (like calcium and iron) at home. Just because supplements are not on a patient's medication profile does not mean they do not take them. A patient who washes down a tetracycline with a calcium supplement or even a (large) glass of milk may completely negate an otherwise brilliant therapeutic plan.

Macrolides and Ketolides

13

Agents: clarithromycin, azithromycin, erythromycin, telithromycin (a ketolide)

Macrolides are among the antibiotics used most frequently in the outpatient setting because of their broad coverage of respiratory pathogens. Though their coverage is broad, it is not particularly deep, because there is increasing resistance to these agents (especially in *Streptococcus pneumoniae*). To combat this resistance, the ketolide derivatives (including telithromycin) have been introduced with better coverage of resistant *S. pneumoniae*. Unfortunately, telithromycin appears to have a significant risk of hepatotoxicity. Although erythromycin is the class patriarch, because of its adverse effects, drug interactions, and frequent dosing, it has little use except as a GI stimulant.

Mechanism of Action

Macrolides and ketolides bind to the 50S subunit of bacterial ribosomes, preventing the ribosomes from shuffling along and adding a new amino acid to the elongating protein chain.

Spectrum

Good: atypicals, *Haemophilus influenzae, Moraxella catarrhalis, Helicobacter pylori, Mycobacterium avium*

Moderate: *S. pneumoniae* (telithromycin > macrolides), *Streptococcus pyogenes*

Poor: staphylococci, enteric GNRs (azithromycin > clarithromycin), anaerobes, enterococci

Adverse Effects

Gastrointestinal: Significant GI adverse effects (nausea, vomiting, diarrhea) have been associated with the macrolides. Erythromycin is the worst offender—it is employed as a prokinetic agent for patients with impaired GI motility.

Hepatic: Rare but serious adverse hepatic events have been associated with the macrolides. Telithromycin has been associated with hepatic failure leading to death or the need for transplantation.

Cardiac: Prolongation of the QT interval has been seen with the macrolides, again most commonly with erythromycin. Use with caution in patients with preexisting heart conditions, those on antiarrhythmic drugs, or those taking interacting drugs (see next section).

Important Facts

- ***Drug interaction alert!*** These drugs (with the exception of azithromycin) are potent inhibitors of drug-metabolizing cytochrome P450 enzymes. Be sure to screen your patient's regimen before starting these agents.

- Azithromycin has a prolonged half-life such that a short course may be adequate for most infections. This makes use of the Z-pak and the extended-release, single-dose Z-max possible.
- Macrolides are bacteriostatic drugs and are not appropriate for infections in which cidal activity is usually required (meningitis, endocarditis, etc.).
- Prevpac is a combination of drugs prescribed for eradication of *H. pylori* and the treatment of peptic ulcer disease. In addition to clarithromycin and lansoprazole, it contains amoxicillin. Be sure to screen patients for both beta-lactam allergies and drug interactions before administering it.
- The spectrum of activity of macrolides makes them an ideal choice for the treatment of community-acquired pneumonia, but the high rates of resistance in *S. pneumoniae* make them risky choices as monotherapy for patients with an infection that is any worse than mild. Treat your more fragile patients with something else, or add a beta-lactam active against *S. pneumoniae*.

What They're Good For

Upper and lower respiratory tract infections, chlamydia, atypical mycobacterial infections, and traveler's diarrhea (azithromycin). Clarithromycin is a key component in the treatment of *H. pylori*–induced GI ulcer disease in combination with other drugs and acid-suppressive agents.

Don't Forget!

Sure, macrolides are good respiratory tract drugs and are relatively benign, but do you really need to be treating your patient's nonspecific (possibly viral) cough and cold with any antibiotic? Besides causing possible adverse reactions and wallet toxicity, overuse of these drugs has contributed to increasing resistance. How about some decongestants, acetaminophen, and chicken soup instead?

14

Oxazolidinones

With the introduction of tedizolid, there are now two oxazolidinones. They share many characteristics, including broad Gram-positive activity and excellent oral bioavailability. Differences between the agents appear to be minor, though linezolid is dosed twice daily and tedizolid is once daily. Linezolid has been on the market for longer and has an advantage over other agents active against MRSA in its clinical trial data supporting its use for MRSA pneumonia.

Mechanism of Action

Oxazolidenones are protein synthesis inhibitors that bind to the 50S ribosomal subunit, blocking the formation of a stable 70S initiation complex and preventing translation. This binding site is distinct from other protein synthesis inhibitors.

Spectrum

Good: MSSA, MRSA, streptococci (including multidrug-resistant *Streptococcus pneumoniae*), enterococci (including VRE), *Nocardia*

Moderate: some atypicals, *Mycobacterium tuberculosis*

Poor: all Gram-negatives, anaerobes

Adverse Effects

Both drugs are generally well tolerated, but they can cause bone marrow suppression, most commonly thrombocytopenia. Bone marrow suppression tends to occur after 2 or more weeks with linezolid therapy and warrants monitoring. Tedizolid seems to have the same effects, though studies of longer duration are limited. With linezolid, it is known that peripheral neuropathy or lactic acidosis may occur after even more prolonged therapy (months) because of toxicity to mitochondria.

Important Facts

- Linezolid and tedizolid have bioavailability of over 90% and oral formulations that greatly increases their utility.
- Linezolid is an inhibitor of monoamine oxidase (MAO) and can cause serotonin syndrome when given concurrently with serotonergic agents such as selective serotonin reuptake inhibitors (SSRIs)—avoid concurrent use if possible. Recent evidence has shown this reaction to be uncommon, but it does occur. Animal models have shown tedizolid to have minimal if any MAO inhibition but human data is limited.
- Linezolid has dual hepatic and renal elimination, and doses do not need to be adjusted in cases of renal or hepatic dysfunction. Tedizolid is eliminated primarily by the liver and may not be sufficiently concentrated in the urine to treat UTIs.
- Tedizolid was studied as a 6-day therapy for skin and skin structure infections and was

comparable to 10 days of linezolid. The short course is nice, but it is possible that shorter courses would work with other drugs too.

- Linezolid has historically been very expensive but recently became generic and prices should drop substantially. Either way, oral formulations are less expensive and more convenient than home-infusion vancomycin and a nurse.

What They're Good For

Infections caused by resistant Gram-positive organisms such as MRSA and VRE. Linezolid is useful for pneumonia, skin and skin structure infections, UTIs, and other uses. Tedizolid is currently only indicated for skin and skin structure infections but may be useful for other types.

Don't Forget!

Monitor patients for bone marrow suppression, particularly during long-term therapy. Avoid concurrent serotonergic drug use with linezolid, if possible. Remember that many SSRIs have long half-lives, so simply discontinuing SSRI use does not avoid a potential interaction. Monitor patients for signs and symptoms of serotonin syndrome if the interaction cannot be avoided.

15

Nitroimidazoles

Nitroimidazoles are around to clean up organisms that the big drug classes—penicillins, cephalosporins, fluoroquinolones, macrolides, etc.—for the most part miss. Worried about gut anaerobes? Metronidazole is there for you. Thinking about parasites in your patient with diarrhea? Try metronidazole or its cousin tinidazole, which has a spectrum of activity similar to that of metronidazole but is approved only for parasitic infections. And of course, if you have gone overboard with the antibiotics and your patient has (mild) *Clostridium difficile* colitis, turn to metronidazole. Just remember the limitations of these drugs: they do not have adequate activity against aerobic bacteria—staphylococci, streptococci, *Escherichia coli*, and such.

Mechanism of Action

Anaerobic bacteria and protozoa—but not aerobic bacteria—activate a part of the nitroimidazole molecule that forms free radicals, which are thought to damage DNA and lead to cell death.

Spectrum: metronidazole

Good: Gram-negative and Gram-positive anaerobes, including *Bacteroides, Fusobacterium*, and *Clostridium* species; protozoa, including *Trichomonas, Entamoeba,* and *Giardia*

Moderate: Helicobacter pylori

Poor: aerobic anything, anaerobes that reside in the mouth (*Peptostreptococcus, Actinomyces, Propionibacterium*)

Adverse Effects

Gastrointestinal: Nausea, vomiting, and diarrhea, along with a metallic taste, are not uncommon with metronidazole. More severe adverse reactions such as hepatitis and pancreatitis are rare.

Neurologic: Dose-related, reversible peripheral neuropathy is occasionally reported with metronidazole, as have very rare cases of confusion and seizures.

Important Facts

- Metronidazole has a reputation for causing a disulfiram-like reaction with the consumption of alcohol, because of its inhibition of aldehyde dehydrogenase. It is prudent to have patients abstain from alcohol while taking metronidazole. Much more concerning is the interaction with warfarin, whose anticoagulant properties are significantly potentiated by inhibition of warfarin metabolism. Careful monitoring is required, and warfarin dose reduction is likely to be necessary.

- Metronidazole has excellent (~100%) bioavailability and none of the drug-chelating concerns of the fluoroquinolones; thus, patients should be switched from IV to oral metronidazole as soon as they are tolerating oral medications.
- Resistance to metronidazole among isolates of *C. difficile* is uncommon, but treatment failure with this infection is not. The organism can exist as an antibiotic-resistant spore and cause relapses after the end of treatment. Patients with moderate to severe *C. difficile* infection, or with more than one relapse of mild disease, should be treated with oral vancomycin or fidaxomicin.

What They're Good For

Infections with documented or suspected abdominal anaerobic bacteria, with adjunctive coverage of aerobes by a second drug when necessary. They are also used for treatment of vaginal trichomoniasis and GI infections caused by susceptible protozoa (amebiasis, giardiasis, etc.). Metronidazole is also a component of therapy for *H. pylori* GI ulcer disease in combination with other antibacterials and acid-suppressive drugs. It is also a treatment option for mild to moderate *C. difficile* infections.

Don't Forget!

The GI flora of humans is a delicate ecosystem—disturb it at your patient's peril. Metronidazole's effect on the normal (primarily anaerobic) GI flora can set up your patients for colonization with nasty bugs such as VRE; determine whether you really need anaerobic coverage.

Nitrofurans and Fosfomycin

16

157 of 368

Agents: nitrofurantoin, fosfomycin

With the rise in resistance among common urinary tract pathogens (primarily *Escherichia coli*), first among TMP/SMX and more recently among the fluoroquinolones, clinicians are left searching for an alternative to treat their patients with uncomplicated cystitis. Nitrofurantoin and fosfomycin, although structurally dissimilar with different mechanisms of action, are two agents that have similar clinical niches. They have retained excellent activity against *E. coli* (> 90% in most studies) and also have adequate coverage of other common community-acquired urinary tract pathogens. Their utility is limited to infections of the lower urinary tract, however, because of pharmacokinetic limitations. Thus, nitrofurantoin and fosfomycin should not be used for more severe urinary tract infections (UTIs) such as pyelonephritis and urosepsis. Intravenous fosfomycin is available in some other countries and used for more severe GNR infections, but since it is unfortunately not presently available in the United States we will not cover it here.

Mechanism of Action

Fosfomycin inhibits bacterial cell wall synthesis in a different way from beta-lactams and glycopeptides, preventing the production of the building blocks of peptidoglycan. The mechanism of action of nitrofurantoin is not well-characterized.

Spectrum

Good: E. coli, Staphylococcus saprophyticus

Moderate: Citrobacter, Klebsiella, Proteus, enterococci, *Pseudomonas* (fosfomycin), *Serratia* (fosfomycin)

Poor: Acinetobacter

Adverse Effects

Gastrointestinal: Nausea and vomiting are occasionally reported. Taking the drugs with food may decrease these effects.

Pulmonary: Nitrofurantoin can cause very rare but serious pulmonary toxicity of two forms. First is an acute pneumonitis manifesting as cough, fever, and dyspnea. This form typically resolves soon after drug discontinuation. A chronic pulmonary fibrosis can occur, most commonly with prolonged nitrofurantoin therapy; recovery of lung function is limited after drug discontinuation.

Important Facts

- It bears repeating: nitrofurantoin and fosfomycin are ineffective for infections outside of the lower urinary tract in the formulations available in the United States. The drugs require high concentrations for antimicrobial activity, and these are reached only where they concentrate in the urine. *Note:* this also means that in patients who have significant renal dysfunction (e.g., a creatinine clearance of less than

50 ml/min), there may be insufficient accumulation of the drug in the urine for activity. Nitrofurantoin in particular should be avoided in these patients.

- Nitrofurantoin comes in two formulations: a crystalline form (Macrodantin) and a macrocrystalline/monohydrate form (Macrobid). The former is dosed four times daily, the latter BID. Guess which one patients prefer? Fosfomycin is only available in the United States as a powder that patients add to water before taking.

- A study of nitrofurantoin showed that it can be used for 5 days instead of the traditional 7-day regimen. This shorter regimen may make nitrofurantoin therapy more palatable for patients who are used to 3-day courses of other UTI drugs (TMP/SMX and fluoroquinolones). Fosfomycin is used for an even shorter duration: its approved regimen for treatment of uncomplicated cystitis is a single dose.

What It's Good For

Treatment of uncomplicated cystitis in patients with adequate renal function (for nitrofurantoin and fosfomycin) and prophylaxis against recurrent uncomplicated lower UTI (for nitrofurantoin).

Don't Forget!

To repeat: do not use these drugs in anything but cystitis. Nitrofurantoin or fosfomycin use in pyelonephritis or urosepsis is a treatment failure waiting to happen.

17

Streptogramins

The increase in resistance to antibiotics among staphylococci and enterococci led to pharmaceutical companies increasing the development of drugs to combat these resistant infections. One of the first of the newer drugs to treat VRE and MRSA infections was quinupristin/dalfopristin. These drugs are two different streptogramins given in a combined formulation. Though each separate streptogramin is bacteriostatic, when given together they act *syner*gistically to give bacter*icid*al activity against some Gram-positive cocci; hence the brand name of this drug: Synercid. Quinupristin/dalfopristin initially enjoyed frequent use, particularly to treat VRE infections, but its use has lessened as other agents have come on the market. Other streptogramins have been developed and are used in animals as growth promoters, a questionable but common practice in modern agriculture (where > 50% of U.S. antibiotics are used).

Mechanism of Action

Quinupristin and dalfopristin bind to different sites on the 50S subunit of the bacterial ribosome to prevent bacterial protein synthesis.

Spectrum

Good: MSSA, MRSA, streptococci, *Enterococcus faecium* (including vancomycin-resistant strains)

Poor: Enterococcus faecalis, anything Gram-negative

Adverse Effects

Quinupristin/dalfopristin can cause phlebitis and ideally should be administered via a central line. It is also associated with a high incidence of myalgias and arthralgias that can limit tolerance to therapy. Quinupristin/dalfopristin also inhibits cytochrome P450 3A4, so clinicians need to be aware of potential drug interactions.

▦ Important Facts

- Quinupristin/dalfopristin must be mixed and administered with 5% dextrose in water (D5W) solutions only. When mixed with normal saline, the drug becomes insoluble and can crystallize, even when a patient's IV line is flushed with saline. Be sure that your patient's nurses know how to flush the line with D5W or another saline-free diluent. The drug is not available orally.
- The arthralgias and myalgias associated with quinupristin/dalfopristin are significant and should not be underestimated. It may be possible to decrease their severity by decreasing the dose, but this could compromise efficacy.
- The indication for the treatment of vancomycin-resistant *E. faecium* infections was removed from the labeling of quinuprisin/dalfopristin due to a lack of follow-up data after the initial

approval. It is no longer considered a first-line therapy for VRE infections.

What It's Good For

Infections caused by MRSA or *E. faecium* in patients not responding to or intolerant of other medications.

Don't Forget!

Quinupristin/dalfopristin is not active against *E. faecalis*. Between the two most common clinical species of *Enterococcus* (*E. faecalis* and *E. faecium*), *E. faecalis* is more common in most hospitals, but it is less likely to be resistant to vancomycin. For this reason, quinupristin/dalfopristin is better employed as a definitive therapy than an empiric one for enterococci unless you strongly suspect *E. faecium* infection. Linezolid and daptomycin do not have this issue and are generally better therapy options.

18

Cyclic Lipopeptides

Agent: daptomycin

Daptomycin is the only cyclic lipopeptide that has made its way onto the market. It has a unique mechanism of action and target compared with other antibiotics. Daptomycin binds to the cell membrane of Gram-positive bacteria, weakening it and allowing essential ions to leak out of the organism. This leads to a rapid depolarization of the membrane potential and cessation of needed cell processes, leading to cell death. Interestingly, instead of blowing the bacteria apart as beta-lactams do, daptomycin leaves the dead bacteria intact.

Mechanism of Action

Daptomycin inserts into the cell membrane of Gram-positive organisms, leading to the leakage of intracellular cations that maintain membrane polarization. The result is rapid depolarization and cell death.

Spectrum

Good: MSSA, MRSA, streptococci
Moderate to Good: enterococci, including VRE
Poor: anything Gram-negative

Adverse Effects

Daptomycin has effects on skeletal muscle that can manifest as muscle pain or weakness, or possibly rhabdomyolysis. To monitor for this effect, creatine kinase (CK) concentrations should be checked weekly while on therapy. This toxicity can be decreased by administering the drug no more than once daily and by adjusting the interval in renal dysfunction. Eosinophilic pneumonia has been reported in patients on daptomycin therapy.

Important Facts

- Daptomycin is active against many resistant Gram-positive organisms, including VRE and MRSA. It has been proven effective in staphylococcal endocarditis (specifically right-sided endocarditis), an indication that few antibiotics have.

- Resistance to daptomycin is uncommon, but it is reported. Before using daptomycin for your patient, ensure that the lab tests the isolate for daptomycin susceptibility. Because a standard MIC for resistance has not yet been defined, labs may report isolates as "nonsusceptible" or, worse, not report them at all if they do not fall into the susceptible range. Ask your lab for specifics on its procedures.

- Though it penetrates lung tissue very well, daptomycin cannot be used to treat pneumonia. Human pulmonary surfactant binds to daptomycin, rendering it inactive. Early clinical trials showed poor outcomes in daptomycin-treated pneumonia patients.

- Daptomycin's FDA-approved dosing is 4–6 mg/kg/day. Several studies suggest that higher doses than this range may be more effective without causing substantially more toxicity. Thus, although we can't necessarily recommend it here, you may see doses as high as 12 mg/kg/day in clinical practice used in difficult-to-treat infections.
- Some studies have shown synergism between daptomycin and some beta-lactams, even in beta-lactam–resistant organisms like MRSA and VRE. It may seem like a weird combination, but there is a logical mechanism behind it that we will explain in our next text, *Antibiotics Complexified.*

What It's Good For

Skin and skin structure infections caused by resistant Gram-positive organisms and staphylococcal bacteremia, including right-sided endocarditis. Daptomycin also has utility in enterococcal bacteremia, though it is not indicated or as well-studied for this use.

Don't Forget!

Monitor CK concentrations and renal function for patients taking daptomycin, particularly if they are on other drugs toxic to skeletal muscle, like HMG-CoA reductase inhibitors.

19

Folate Antagonists

The combination drug TMP/SMX is the most widely used folate antagonist, active against both bacterial and parasitic/fungal infections. TMP/SMX was once considered a broad-spectrum antibacterial drug that has since fallen victim to the relentless march of antibiotic resistance; however, it is still a drug of choice for a number of indications. Resistance varies considerably by geographic region, so consider your local antibiogram before using TMP/SMX as empiric therapy. The other agents are used against parasitic/fungal infections. The information below refers to TMP/SMX except where noted.

Mechanism of Action

These drugs inhibit steps in the folate biosynthesis pathway, depleting the pool of nucleosides and ultimately leading to inhibition of DNA synthesis in susceptible organisms.

Spectrum

Good: Staphylococcus aureus (including many MRSA strains), *Haemophilus influenzae, Stenotrophomonas maltophilia, Listeria, Pneumocystis jirovecii* (formerly known as *P. carinii*), *Toxoplasma gondii* (pyrimethamine and sulfadiazine)

Moderate: enteric GNRs, *Streptococcus pneumoniae*, *Salmonella*, *Shigella*, *Nocardia*, *Streptococcus pyogenes*

Poor: Pseudomonas, enterococci, anaerobes

Adverse Effects

Dermatologic: TMP/SMX frequently causes rash, usually because of the sulfamethoxazole component. Rash is much more common in HIV/AIDS patients. Although these rashes are usually not severe, life-threatening dermatologic reactions such as toxic epidermal necrolysis and Stevens-Johnson syndrome also occur.

Hematologic: A primarily dose-dependent bone-marrow suppression can be seen with TMP/SMX, especially at the higher doses used to treat *Pneumocystis* infections.

Renal: Confusingly, TMP/SMX can cause both true and pseudo-renal failure. Crystalluria and AIN caused by the SMX component can lead to acute renal failure; however, the blockade of creatinine secretion by TMP can cause an increase in serum creatinine without a true decline in glomerular filtration rate. TMP can also cause hyperkalemia in a fashion similar to the potassium-sparing diuretics (e.g., triamterene).

Important Facts

* For years, TMP/SMX was standard first-line therapy for treatment of acute uncomplicated

cystitis in women. Guidelines suggest, however, that in areas with local resistance rates greater than 15–20% in *Escherichia coli*, an alternative drug (e.g., nitrofurantoin) should be used. At a minimum TMP/SMX should not be used for empiric therapy of complicated UTI (pyelonephritis or urosepsis).

- TMP/SMX comes in a fixed 1:5 ratio of the two components. Dosing is based on the TMP component. The oral tablet comes in two strengths: single-strength (80:400 mg TMP:SMX) and double-strength (160:800 mg TMP:SMX). TMP/SMX has excellent oral bioavailability, allowing for conversion to oral therapy when patients are tolerating oral medications.

- TMP/SMX has a significant drug interaction with warfarin, leading to higher-than-anticipated prothrombin times. TMP/SMX should be avoided in patients on warfarin if possible. If coadministration is absolutely necessary, careful monitoring of the patient's international normalized ratio is required.

- TMP/SMX is fairly insoluble in IV solutions, and relatively large volumes of diluent are needed for it to go into solution. Be aware that this fluid may be considerable, particularly for volume-overloaded patients such as those with heart failure.

- The predominant strain of MRSA that causes outpatient MRSA infections is very susceptible to TMP/SMX. This strain likes to cause skin infections with abscesses, often large ones. TMP/SMX is a good choice of therapy for staphylococcal skin infections, but abscesses must be drained.

What They're Good For

Treatment of uncomplicated lower UTIs (empirically in areas with low local resistance, definitively whenever susceptible), prophylaxis against recurrent UTIs, treatment of listeria meningitis, treatment of and prophylaxis for *P. jirovecii* pneumonia, and treatment of *Toxoplasma* encephalitis. TMP/SMX is also an alternative therapy for bacterial prostatitis, typhoid fever, and methicillin-resistant *S. aureus* infections. Sulfadiazine is used in the treatment of toxoplasmosis.

Don't Forget!

Patients allergic to TMP/SMX may have cross-reactions to other drugs containing sulfonamide moieties, such as furosemide, sulfadiazine, acetazolamide, hydrochlorothiazide, and glipizide.

20

Lincosamides

Clindamycin can be considered a mix of vancomycin and metronidazole; it has attributes of each drug, but it is not quite as good as either one alone. Clindamycin is an alternative when treatment requires Gram-positive activity (as with beta-lactam allergies), but it has more variable activity than vancomycin against such pathogens as MRSA and *Streptococcus pyogenes*. Clindamycin also covers many anaerobic organisms, but there is a higher level of resistance among the Gram-negative anaerobes (such as *Bacteroides fragilis*) than with metronidazole. Because of these limitations and clindamycin's tendency to cause GI toxicity, it is best used empirically for nonsevere infections of the skin and oral cavity, or as definitive therapy when susceptibilities are known.

Mechanism of Action

Clindamycin binds at a site on the 50S ribosome right next to where the macrolides bind and acts similarly in preventing protein synthesis by preventing the ribosome from moving on to adding another amino acid in the protein chain.

Spectrum: clindamycin

Good: many Gram-positive anaerobes, *Plasmodium* species (malaria), *S. pyogenes*

Moderate: Staphylococcus aureus (including many MRSA), Gram-negative anaerobes, *Chlamydia trachomatis, Pneumocystis jirovecii, Actinomyces, Toxoplasma*

Poor: enterococci, *Clostridium difficile*, Gram-negative aerobes

Adverse Effects

Gastrointestinal: Diarrhea is one of the most common adverse effects associated with clindamycin. Clindamycin itself can cause relatively benign, self-limited diarrhea or can result in more severe diarrhea resulting from superinfection with *C. difficile. C. difficile*–associated diarrhea and colitis can occur during or after clindamycin therapy and can be life-threatening. Patients with diarrhea need evaluation for *C. difficile* disease, especially if it is severe, is associated with fever, or persists after clindamycin therapy.

Dermatologic: Rash may occur with clindamycin, very rarely with severe manifestations such as Stevens-Johnson syndrome.

■ Important Facts

• Clindamycin is a reasonable alternative drug for the treatment of staphylococcal infections; however, care must be taken in interpreting the antibiotic susceptibility of these isolates. A significant proportion of organisms that are reported as clindamycin-susceptible but erythromycin-resistant may harbor a gene for resistance that may lead to high-level clindamycin resistance during therapy. Erythromycin-resistant, clindamycin-susceptible strains should be screened with a D-test (the microbiology lab will know what you mean) before using clindamycin. If the D-test is positive, then inducible clindamycin resistance is present and clindamycin should not be used.

- Clindamycin's inhibition of protein synthesis and activity against organisms in stationary-phase growth has been utilized in the treatment of necrotizing fasciitis and other toxin-mediated diseases. Consider the addition of clindamycin to beta-lactam–based therapy when treating these types of infections.
- Clindamycin is nearly 100% orally bioavailable, but oral doses are generally lower than IV doses in order to improve GI tolerance.
- Many community-acquired MRSA infections are susceptible to clindamycin, but not as many as are susceptible to TMP/SMX.

What It's Good For

Treatment of skin and soft-tissue infections, infections of the oral cavity, and anaerobic intra-abdominal infections. It is used topically in the treatment of acne. Clindamycin is a second-line agent (in combination with primaquine) in the treatment of *P. jirovecii* pneumonia. It is also used to treat malaria in combination with other drugs, to treat bacterial vaginosis, and in the prophylaxis of bacterial endocarditis.

Don't Forget!

Almost all antibiotics have been associated with an increased risk of *C. difficile* disease; however, some studies suggest that clindamycin may confer an especially high risk (note that this is a popular board exam question). Although it is a convenient and relatively well-tolerated drug, clindamycin should not be used lightly because of this risk.

Polymyxins

21

Agents: colistin (colistimethate sodium), polymyxin B

Polymyxins are an older class of antibiotics that had nearly vanished from systemic use years ago in favor of the "safer" aminoglycosides. Unfortunately, the continuous evolution of bacterial resistance has forced the medical community to revisit the use of colistin and polymyxin B in the treatment of resistant Gram-negative infections. This is problematic because these drugs have not been evaluated with the rigor of the modern drug approval process, and pharmacokinetic and efficacy data on their use are limited. However, they have been found to be useful in the treatment of infections caused by highly resistant Gram-negative organisms such as *Acinetobacter baumannii, Pseudomonas aeruginosa,* and carbapenem-resistant Enterobacteriaceae (CRE) such as *Klebsiella pneumoniae*.

Mechanism of Action

Polymyxins bind to the outer membrane of Gram-negative bacteria, leading to disruption of membrane stability and leakage of cellular contents.

Spectrum

Good: many GNRs, including multidrug resistant *A. baumannii*, *P. aeruginosa*, and *K. pneumoniae*

Moderate: Stenotrophomonas maltophilia

Poor: all Gram-positive organisms, anaerobes, *Proteus, Providencia, Burkholderia, Serratia*, and Gram-negative cocci

Adverse Effects

Renal: The most common adverse effect is nephrotoxicity due to acute tubular necrosis. Acute kidney injury commonly occurs in clinical use, though the incidence of polymyxin-induced toxicity is hard to estimate because most recent studies of polymyxins are noncomparative evaluations of salvage therapies in very ill patients. Several studies suggest that polymyxin B is less nephrotoxic than colistin. Avoid concomitant nephrotoxins if possible.

Neurological: Neurotoxicity is less common. It can manifest as dizziness, weakness, paresthesias, or mental status changes. Neuromuscular blockade can also occur and may lead to fatal respiratory arrest.

Important Facts

- Colistin and polymyxin B are very similar drugs. Colistin may be more active, but to be given systemically it is administered as colistimethate sodium. Colistimethate is then converted into active colistin in the body. Colistimethate is renally cleared, and only the proportion that is not cleared is converted to colistin. In the United States, it is typically dosed as milligrams of "colistin base activity" (~400 mg colistimethate = 150 mg of colistin base activity), though the actual amount that is systemically active differs in each patient. Colistin itself is not used systemically. When most references refer to "colistin" (including this one), they are referring to "colistimethate sodium."

- One area where polymyxins differ is in pharmacokinetics. As mentioned above, colistin is given as a renally eliminated prodrug. Polymyxin B is given in its active form and has more predictable pharmacokinetics. Both drugs should be given with loading doses.
- Polymyxin B is not eliminated renally and modern pharmacokinetic studies suggest that it should not be dose adjusted in renal dysfunction. It is unlikely to be successful in treating urinary tract infections (UTIs).
- To further confound colistin use, different standards of dosing are used by different countries. The U.S. formulation is dosed in milligrams of colistin base activity, while Europe and many other parts of the world dose in international units. When comparing, it is important to know that 1 mg of colistin base activity is equivalent to about 30,000 units. It actually calculates to ~33,333 units, but many references round this number.
- Two ways of summarizing colistin dosing:
  - 1,000,000 units ≈ 80 mg colistimethate ≈ 30 mg colistin base activity
  - 1 mg colistin base activity ≈ 2.7 mg colistimethate ≈ 30,000 units

- Never prescribe or recommend colistin doses in terms of mg of colistimethate. A misinterpretation can be fatal.
- Speaking of confounding dosing standards, polymyxin B is dosed in either milligrams or international units. Note that 1 mg = 10,000 units.
- Because polymyxin drugs are generally last-line antibiotics, they are frequently used in combination with other drugs. Various combinations of colistin and other drugs such as rifampin and meropenem may be better than colistin use alone; this is an area of active study.
- The oral formulation of colistin is given only for bowel decontamination, such as before GI surgery. Don't try to convert someone from IV to PO colistin to treat a systemic infection.
- Aerosolized polymyxins are used to decrease colonization with Gram-negative bacteria (principally *Pseudomonas*) in some patients, particularly those with cystic fibrosis. They should be prepared just before administration. Some experts have used aerosolized drugs to treat pneumonia also, though evidence for this practice is not yet very strong.

What They're Good For

Polymyxins are useful in the treatment of multidrug-resistant Gram-negative infections including pneumonia, bacteremia, sepsis, and complicated UTIs. Because polymyxins are poorly studied in many of these disease states, other drugs should be used if pathogens are susceptible.

Don't Forget!

While estimates of polymyxin nephrotoxicity vary, the incidence is substantial, particularly in critically ill patients who may not be able to tolerate the renal insult. Monitor renal function closely in patients receiving polymyxins and avoid other nephrotoxins if possible, including vancomycin.

22

Fidaxomicin

Agent: fidaxomicin

Fidaxomicin is a new addition to the antibiotic armamentarium that has one use: the treatment of *Clostridium difficile* infections. It is a nonabsorbed macrocyclic antibiotic with a narrow spectrum that is ideal for treating infections caused by *C. difficile* because it is sparing to the normal flora of the GI tract, allowing it to be restored during therapy.

Mechanism of Action

Fidaxomicin is a ribosomal protein synthesis inhibitor that is bactericidal. It is classified as a macrolide by the U.S. FDA but, unlike other macrolides, is not absorbed in the GI tract and is able to kill susceptible organisms.

Spectrum

Good: C. difficile
Poor: anything else, including *Bacteroides* species and enteric GNRs

Adverse Effects

As a nonabsorbed antibiotic, fidaxomicin would be expected to have few systemic adverse effects. Most of the adverse effects reported in clinical trials are associated with *C. difficile* infection, including nausea, diarrhea, abdominal pain, and cramping. More experience is needed to further classify the adverse reactions with fidaxomicin.

Important Facts

- In a clinical trial comparing it with vancomycin capsules, fidaxomicin showed similar clinical efficacy to oral vancomycin. However, it was superior in preventing recurrences of *C. difficile* infection and may be preferred for patients at high risk of recurrence.
- The advantages of fidaxomicin in sparing the normal flora of the GI tract are likely negated when it is coadministered with oral vancomycin or metronidazole. Two drugs are not always better than one, and these combinations should probably be avoided.
- Currently, fidaxomicin is expensive. Patient assistance programs are available to help acquire the drug for those who need it. The high cost of the drug is cheaper than an admission for *C. difficile* relapse, but determining who the best candidates for fidaxomicin use is a challenge.

What It's Good For

Clostridium difficile infections, ranging from diarrhea to pseudomembranous colitis.

Don't Forget!

Fidaxomicin has an important benefit in lowering *C. difficile* infection recurrence, but its cost necessitates careful determination of which patients are most likely to benefit from it.

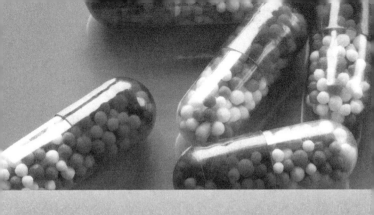

Antimycobacterial Drugs

PART 3

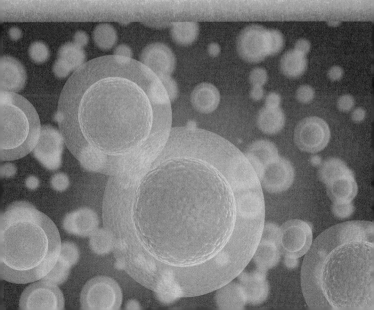

23

Antimycobacterial Drugs

Introduction to Antimycobacterial Drugs

Tuberculosis, the disease caused by *Mycobacterium tuberculosis*, is one of the world's most formidable infections. Tuberculosis and other mycobacterial diseases are difficult to treat for several reasons. Mycobacteria replicate more slowly than "typical" bacteria such as *Escherichia coli* or *Staphylococcus aureus*. This may seem to make the disease easier to control, but it makes pharmacotherapy more difficult because rapidly dividing cells are most metabolically active and therefore susceptible to antibiotic chemotherapy.

Mycobacteria can also exist in a dormant state, making them resistant to nearly all antibiotics. In the host, they live inside human cells, and therefore antimicrobials that have poor intracellular penetration are ineffective. Mycobacteria also have cell walls that are structurally different from typical Gram-positive and Gram-negative bacteria. The outermost layer of mycobacteria consists of phospholipids and mycolic acids that make a waxy layer that resists penetration from antibiotics. Arabinogalactan and peptidoglycan are polysaccharide components of the cell wall, but the peptidoglycan is not accessible to beta-lactam antibiotics, and

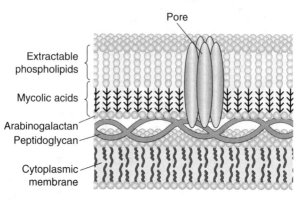

Mycobacterial Cell Wall

they are poorly active. Figure 23–1 shows the basic structure of mycobacteria.

The pharmacotherapy of mycobacterial disease is complex. Combinations of drugs are always given for patients with active disease to minimize the development of resistance and shorten the duration of therapy. These combinations frequently have pharmacokinetic drug interactions with both each other and other medications that the patient is on (in part because immunocompromised patients are particularly vulnerable to mycobacterial disease and they tend to be on drugs with many interactions). Because mycobacteria grow slowly, standard susceptibility testing takes weeks instead of days to perform, so empiric regimens are often given for extended durations. For tuberculosis, the standard of care for patients with active infections is to start with a four-drug regimen, so compliance and careful watching for drug interactions are important.

First-line drugs for tuberculosis and *Mycobacterium avium–intracellulare* complex (MAC) are discussed in this section. Many second-line drugs are available for tuberculosis; however, because the treatment of multidrug-resistant tuberculosis (MDR-TB) requires the management of an infectious diseases specialist, we omit them from this text—there is nothing "simplified" about MDR-TB. The following antimycobacterial drugs are listed in the antibacterial chapters: fluoroquinolones (moxifloxacin is particularly active), macrolides, and aminoglycosides. It is particularly important to know the toxicities of the first-line agents for tuberculosis, because they each have a characteristic one. You can expect questions about these characteristics to pop-up on a lot of exams, both in school and for licensure.

24

Rifamycins

The rifamycins are cornerstones of therapy for both tuberculosis and MAC. They are protein synthesis inhibitors that inhibit transcription of DNA to bacterial messenger RNA. Rifampin (or rifampicin, as it is known in European literature) is one of the two most important drugs in tuberculosis pharmacotherapy. The rifamycins are potent inducers of the cytochrome P450 system, and patients receiving them should *always* be screened for drug interactions. In addition to their activity against mycobacteria, rifamycins are active against many "typical" bacteria as well and are sometimes added to other therapies, particularly to treat difficult MRSA infections.

Mechanism of Action

Rifamycins are protein synthesis inhibitors that work by inhibiting RNA polymerase, preventing transcription by blocking the production of messenger RNA. This separates them from other protein synthesis inhibitors, which inhibit translation.

Spectrum

Good: most mycobacteria

Moderate: *Staphylococcus, Acinetobacter,* Enterobacteriaceae

Poor: "typical" bacteria as monotherapy, some very rare mycobacteria

Adverse Effects

Rifamycins are generally well-tolerated drugs that are most notorious for their potent CYP450-inducing effects. Their potent induction of metabolism can lead to subtherapeutic concentrations of other drugs that can manifest with devastating clinical consequences, such as loss of seizure control (anticonvulsants) or organ rejection (antirejection agents). Rifampin characteristically colors secretions (urine, tears, etc.) orange-red and can actually stain contact lenses, which should not be worn during rifampin therapy. Otherwise, this effect is nonpermanent and not harmful, which patients appreciate knowing. Rifamycins can also cause hepatotoxicity. Other side effects include rash, nausea, vomiting, and hypersensitivity (often fever).

Important Facts

- Rifampin is a drug of choice for tuberculosis, while rifabutin is a drug of choice for MAC, although both drugs have activity against both pathogens. MAC infections are most common in patients with HIV, who are often taking antiretroviral therapy that is metabolized by CYP450. Because rifabutin has somewhat less-potent CYP450-inducing effects than rifampin, it is more commonly used in MAC infections to minimize the impact of drug interactions in this population.

- Rifampin (or rifabutin) is one of the two most important drugs in the treatment of tuberculosis (the other being isoniazid). If an isolate of *Mycobacterium tuberculosis* is rifampin-resistant, then the likelihood of successful pharmacotherapy is lower and more complicated regimens must be used for a longer duration.

- All systemic rifamycins induce CYP450 enzymes and can induce the metabolism of drugs through other hepatic pathways as well. Always screen for drug interactions when starting a rifamycin.

- Rifabutin induces CYP450 metabolism less potently than rifampin does, but it is still a potent inducer and requires careful review of potential consequences of its interaction on a patient's drug regimen.

- Rifapentine is a second-line drug that is given once weekly. It shares susceptibility with rifampin and rifabutin, meaning that if an isolate is resistant to one drug, it is resistant to all of them. Recent guidelines recommend it in combination with isoniazid as a once-weekly therapy for latent tuberculosis.

- Rifaximin is a nonabsorbed rifamycin used only in the treatment or prevention of GI conditions. It is not used for mycobacterial diseases and is listed here only for completeness.

- Rifamycins should not be used as monotherapy for treatment of active tuberculosis, but rifampin can be used as monotherapy to treat latent tuberculosis infection.

What They're Good For

Treatment of active tuberculosis and MAC, in combination with other agents; latent tuberculosis; and selected bacterial infections (most notably bacterial infections involving prosthetic material—such as an artificial hip or heart valve—in combination with standard antibacterials).

Don't Forget!

Ensure that patients are informed that their urine and other secretions may turn orange or red. That's a surprise that most people don't want and could lead to completely unnecessary Emergency Room visits!

25

Isoniazid

Isoniazid is active only against *Mycobacterium tuberculosis* and the related *Mycobacterium kansasii*, but it is one of the two most important drugs in tuberculosis pharmacotherapy (the other being rifampin), being effective against both actively growing and dormant mycobacteria. It is used in the treatment of both active and latent tuberculosis.

Mechanism of Action

Isoniazid prevents the synthesis of mycolic acids in the cell wall by inhibiting enzymes that catalyze their production.

Spectrum

Active only against *M. tuberculosis* and *M. kansasii*.

Adverse Effects

Like several other tuberculosis medications, hepatotoxicity is a concern. Many patients will experience asymptomatic elevations in liver transaminases early in therapy. In most cases, these will resolve on their own and the patient can complete treatment. However, if the enzyme levels are many times the upper limit of normal and/or the patient experience symptoms of hepatitis (nausea, abdominal pain, jaundice), the drug needs to be stopped to prevent severe liver damage. Isoniazid's other characteristic adverse reaction is peripheral neuropathy. This can be prevented by administering pyridoxine (vitamin B_6), which is recommended for patients at risk for developing neuropathy (e.g., diabetics, pregnant women, alcohol abusers). Other neurotoxicities that are less common include opticneuritis and, rarely, seizures. Drug-induced lupus can also occur; this abates with the cessation of therapy. Hypersensitivity can be seen, most commonly as rash or drug fever.

Important Facts

- Isoniazid is a drug of choice for the treatment of latent tuberculosis. It can be given as monotherapy for latent disease because the burden of organisms is much lower than in active tuberculosis, where resistance can develop to monotherapy.
- Isoniazid is a classic example of a drug with variable pharmacogenomic metabolism. "Rapid acetylators" of isoniazid metabolize it more quickly than "slow acetylators," but the clinical significance of this is unknown. Genetic testing is not routinely performed before starting isoniazid.
- Isoniazid is bactericidal against growing mycobacteria, but bacteriostatic against dormant mycobacteria.
- Patients should be advised not to drink alcohol while taking isoniazid. This has nothing to do with the common myth that alcohol decreases

antibiotic effectiveness; it is to prevent an additive risk of hepatotoxicity.

What It's Good For

Isoniazid is a drug of choice for both active and latent tuberculosis. For treatment of active tuberculosis, it must be combined with other medications. The combination of isoniazid and rifampin is recommended for the consolidation phase of non-MDR-TB.

Don't Forget!

Although guidelines recommend adding pyridoxine for preventing neuropathy only in high-risk patients, there's no downside in recommending it to all your patients receiving isoniazid. Don't confuse pyridoxine with pyrazinamide (discussed in the next section) and assume that your patient is receiving both drugs when he or she is not. Most patients with tuberculosis should be taking both pyridoxine and pyrazinamide during the initial phase of therapy.

26

Pyrazinamide

Agent: pyrazinamide

Pyrazinamide is a first-line drug for the treatment of tuberculosis. As part of the initial four-drug regimen for active tuberculosis, it enables the overall duration of therapy to be shortened from 9 months to 6 months. Pyrazinamide has bactericidal activity against even slow-growing *Mycobacterium tuberculosis*. It is generally used only in the first 2 months of tuberculosis therapy.

Mechanism of Action

Pyrazinamide is a prodrug with an unclear mechanism of action. In its active forms it is thought to prevent the production of mycolic acids by inhibiting the enzyme fatty acid synthetase I, though it likely has other effects as well.

Spectrum

Active only against *M. tuberculosis*.

Adverse Effects

The key adverse effects for pyrazinamide are hyperuricemia and hepatotoxicity. Hepatotoxicity (chiefly hepatitis) is dose-dependent and less common at the lower doses given today than the higher ones previously used. Hyperuricemia is predictable and can rarely precipitate gout, leading to withdrawal of pyrazinamide from the regimen and an extension of the duration of tuberculosis therapy. Arthralgias also occur and are separate from hyperuricemia; these can be managed with over-the-counter pain medications.

Important Facts

- Interestingly, pyrazinamide is active only in acidic environments (pH< 6). This would be problematic for some diseases, but it is perfect for the caseous granulomas that active tuberculosis forms. It also works intracellularly in phagocytes.
- Be careful not to confuse this drug with pyridoxine, which most patients with active tuberculosis should also be taking to prevent isoniazid-induced peripheral neuropathy.

What It's Good For

Pyrazinamide's only use is in the initial phase of active tuberculosis treatment.

Don't Forget!

Tell your patients to report any signs of hepatitis (dark urine, abdominal pain, loss of appetite) when they are on pyrazinamide or any first-line tuberculosis therapy.

Ethambutol

27

Ethambutol is a first-line drug for the treatment of both active tuberculosis and MAC infections. Like pyrazinamide, ethambutol is principally used in the initial four-drug phase of active tuberculosis, but it is usually given for the duration of MAC therapy.

Mechanism of Action

Ethambutol inhibits the enzyme aribinosyl transferase III, which blocks production of arabinogalactan. Because arabinogalactan is a component of the cell wall of mycobacteria but not "typical" bacteria, the microbial activity of ethambutol is limited to mycobacteria.

Spectrum

Mycobacterium tuberculosis, *Mycobacterium avium–intracellulare* complex, *Mycobacterium kansasii*

Adverse Effects

The characteristic adverse effect of ethambutol is optic neuritis, often manifesting as decreased visual acuity or the inability to differentiate red from green. It is dependent on both the dose and duration of therapy and is generally reversible; monitoring is required to detect this problem. Use of ethambutol in children younger than 5 years old is not recommended, because they are generally not able to reliably perform the vision tests needed for monitoring. Rash and drug fever occur uncommonly.

Important Facts

- Ethambutol is very well tolerated, and it is the one component of the "RIPE" (**R**ifampin, **I**sonizid, **P**yrazinamide, **E**thambutol) active tuberculosis regimen that is not associated with hepatotoxicity.
- Ethambutol can be used as a substitute for rifampin in patients who are unable to take that medication during the continuation phase (after 2 months) of active tuberculosis therapy. However, the duration of therapy has to be extended relative to what it would be with rifampin and isoniazid.
- Ethambutol is one of the primary first-line drugs (along with a macrolide and rifabutin) for treating MAC infections.

What It's Good For

First-line therapy for both active tuberculosis and MAC infections. Second-line therapy in patients unable to tolerate rifampin during the continuation phase.

Don't Forget!

Want an easy way to remember that ethambutol causes optic neuritis? Just remember: for **E**thambutol, the **E**yes have it!

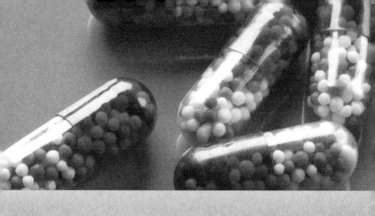

Antifungal Drugs

PART 4

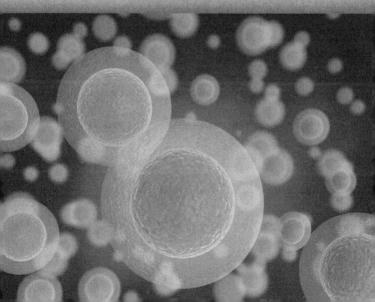

28

Antifungal Drugs

Introduction to Antifungal Drugs

Fungi rule their own kingdom. There are possibly millions of species of these saprophytic and parasitic organisms, but, as with bacteria, only a small minority are pathogens. Most pathogenic fungi are opportunistic and require a compromised host or disrupted barrier in order to cause infection in humans. In a way, the increase of systemic fungal infections can be seen as a medical advance, because improvements in transplantation, oncology, rheumatology, neonatology, geriatrics, and other fields have created more susceptible hosts for fungi. The practice of medical mycology has expanded greatly.

Microscopic fungi exist in two basic forms: yeasts and molds. Table 28–1 highlights some of the medically important fungi. Yeasts are unicellular forms of fungi that reproduce by budding. When they are left to grow in colonies, they have a moist, shiny appearance. Molds are multicellular fungi that consist of many branching hyphae and can reproduce either by translocation of existing hyphae to a new area, or through spore formation and spread (hence, one bad apple really does spoil a bunch). They have a familiar fuzzy appearance, such as the *Rhizopus* that you have undoubtedly seen on bread.

TABLE 28–1
Common Clinical Fungi

Yeasts	Dimorphic Fungi	Molds
Candida	Histoplasma	Aspergillus
Cryptococcus	Blastomyces	Fusarium
	Coccidioides	Scedosporium
	Paracoccidioides	Mucorales

In addition to these two basic forms, there are dimorphic fungi that can exist in either form. These fungi are often mold-like at room temperature, but yeast-like at body temperature. They are frequently referred to as "endemic" fungi, because they cause infections endemic to certain regions of the world; for example, *Coccidioides immitis* causes an infection in the southwestern United States and central California that is sometimes called valley fever.

Yeasts, particularly *Candida* species, have become a leading cause of nosocomial bloodstream infections. This makes them important infectious agents that are worthy of our attention. Unfortunately, invasive *Candida* infections are challenging to diagnose: the presence of *Candida* in a culture might represent colonization, not infection (think colonization of urinary catheters). On the other hand, deep-seated *Candida* infections frequently are not detected by standard methods and sometimes only found on autopsy. Molds generally cause invasive disease in immunocompromised hosts, but they should be considered in patients with various levels of immune system suppression, not just those in the most severe category. Dimorphic fungi usually cause mild, self-limited disease, but some can also cause fatal disseminated disease, particularly in patients with suppressed immunity.

Antifungal pharmacotherapy has several problems that often make fungal infections more difficult to treat than bacterial infections. One is that pathogens can be more difficult to isolate on culture than bacterial organisms. This makes the prompt initiation of empiric therapy important when invasive fungal infections are suspected. Prophylaxis may also be used in highly susceptible populations to prevent fungal infections from developing.

Another concern in the treatment of fungal disease is that most centers do not conduct antifungal susceptibility testing. This forces clinicians to guess at likely susceptibility patterns based on speciation rather than test results. Even with the "right" antifungal, the capabilities of the host significantly affect the likelihood of success in treating an invasive fungal infection. For neutropenic patients with mycoses, neutrophil recovery is a significant predictor of success, and patients with a prolonged immunocompromised status have a much worse prognosis. Therefore, while the selection of an appropriate antifungal is important, control of patient-specific factors is equally important to increase the likelihood of success, whether it is the need to remove a central venous catheter or to decrease doses of immunosuppressants.

Compared with the abundance of drugs available to kill bacteria, the number of systemic antifungal drugs is much lower. Selective toxicity is more difficult to achieve with eukaryotic fungi than with prokaryotic bacteria. Several newly marketed agents have changed the way fungal infections are treated. The chapters that follow introduce these agents in more detail.

Polyenes

For many years, amphotericin B deoxycholate was the standard of care for many systemic fungal infections, for both its broad antifungal spectrum and a lack of available alternatives. However, amphotericin B is notable for its toxicities, principally nephrotoxicity and infusion-related reactions. To attenuate these toxicities, three lipid forms were developed: amphotericin B colloidal dispersion (ABCD), amphotericin B lipid complex (ABLC), and liposomal amphotericin B (LAmB).

Amphotericin B formulations have seen considerably less use since the introduction of the echinocandins and broad-spectrum azoles, but they still have utility. Activity against yeasts and many molds, proven efficacy in understudied disease states, and a long history of use help maintain their place in the antifungal armamentarium.

Mechanism of Action

Polyenes such as amphotericin B bind to ergosterol in the fungal cell membrane, forming pores in the membrane and leading to the leakage of cell contents with eventual cell death.

Spectrum

Good: most species of *Candida* and *Aspergillus*, *Cryptococcus neoformans*, dimorphic fungi, many molds

Moderate: Mucorales

Poor: Candida lusitaniae, Aspergillus terreus

Adverse Effects

Infusion-related reactions: Infusion-related reactions with amphotericin B products include fever, chills, and rigors and can be impressive. These symptoms can be attenuated by premedicating with acetaminophen, hydrocortisone, and sometimes other medications. Liposomal amphotericin B has the lowest incidence of infusion-related reactions; amphotericin B colloidal dispersion has the greatest.

Renal: Nephrotoxicity with amphotericin B products is common. Both direct effects on the distal tubule and indirect effects through vasoconstriction of the afferent arteriole cause the nephrotoxicity, and nephrotoxicity also leads to wasting of magnesium and potassium, such that patients frequently need supplementation. All of the lipid formulations have less nephrotoxicity than the conventional amphotericin B deoxycholate formulation; liposomal amphotericin B has the least.

Others: Increased transaminases and rash can occur with amphotericin B products as well.

Dosing Issues

The multiple formulations of amphotericin B can lead to confusion over their dosing. Amphotericin B deoxycholate is generally dosed between 0.5 and

1.5 mg/kg/day, where the lipid formulations are dosed at 3–6 mg/kg/day. Whether the lipid formulations are equivalent with each other is a matter of debate, but most clinicians dose them as if they are. Fatal overdoses of amphotericin B deoxycholate have occurred when dosed as the lipid forms— a 5–3-fold overdose. Mind your formulation.

Important Facts

- Amphotericin B nephrotoxicity can be attenuated by the process of sodium loading: administer boluses of normal saline before and after the amphotericin infusion. Sodium loading is an inexpensive and easy way of protecting the kidneys.
- Many practitioners administer such drugs as acetaminophen, diphenhydramine, and hydrocortisone to decrease the incidence and severity of infusion-related reactions of amphotericin B. Meperidine is often given to treat rigors when they develop, but be wary of using this drug in patients who develop renal dysfunction because it has a neurotoxic metabolite that is eliminated renally.
- Whether differences in efficacy exist between the lipid formulations of amphotericin B is a matter of debate, but differences in safety do exist. In terms of infusion-related reactions, ABCD seems to have the worst, while LAmB has the least. All of them have less nephrotoxicity than amphotericin B deoxycholate, but LAmB seems to have the least of all.
- Nystatin is used only topically due to poor tolerance when given systemically.

What They're Good For

Amphotericin B formulations remain the drugs of choice for cryptococcal meningitis and serious forms of some other fungal infections, such as those caused by dimorphic fungi and some molds. Because of their broad spectrum, they are also a reasonable choice if fungal infection is suspected but the infecting organism is not known, as in febrile neutropenia. Their use in candidiasis and aspergillosis has declined with the availability of newer, safer agents.

Don't Forget!

Double-check that dose of amphotericin B; which formulation are you using?

Agent: flucytosine (5-FC)

Flucytosine was originally investigated as an oncology drug, but it was found to be significantly more active against fungi than against human cancer cells. The primary role of flucytosine is in combination therapy with amphotericin B formulations for cryptococcal disease. Because of its toxicity and relative lack of efficacy, it is rarely used for other infections.

Mechanism of Action

Flucytosine is deaminated inside fungal cells to 5-fluorouracil, which is further converted into metabolites that interfere with both protein and DNA synthesis.

Spectrum

Good: in combination with amphotericin B: *Cryptococcus neoformans*, most species of *Candida*
Moderate: monotherapy: *Cryptococcus neoformans*, most species of *Candida*
Poor: molds, *Candida krusei*

Adverse Effects

Flucytosine, which is also called 5-FC, is fluorouracil for fungi. When this fact is considered, the adverse effects are predictable. Flucytosine is only relatively selective for fungi and can cause considerable bone marrow suppression, particularly in higher doses or during prolonged courses. GI complaints are more common, but they are less severe.

Important Facts

- Drug concentration monitoring is available for flucytosine: check a peak concentration about 2 hours after the dose is given. However, do not rely on flucytosine concentrations alone to monitor for toxicity—hematology values are more important than drug levels. Also, in most hospitals flucytosine levels are a "sendout" lab that can take up to a week to be resulted; given the most common duration of therapy for flucytosine is 2 weeks, the practical utility of flucytosine levels is limited.
- Flucytosine generally should not be used as monotherapy for invasive candidiasis because of the potential emergence of resistance *in vivo*.
- The most common use for flucytosine is in combination with an amphotericin B formulation for cryptococcal meningitis. Though this combination is recommended in guidelines and very common, some clinicians have questioned the value of flucytosine. In an early clinical study for this indication, flucytosine use was associated with more rapid sterility of cerebrospinal fluid cultures but showed no obvious clinical benefit. However, more recent studies have shown a survival benefit with flucytosine use. This is obviously a plus in terms of efficacy, but flucytosine is difficult to obtain or afford in resource-poor countries where HIV infection is highly endemic.

- Flucytosine is commonly abbreviated as 5-FC, but this practice should be avoided because it can be confused with the related 5-FU (fluorouracil), which is considerably more toxic.

What It's Good For

As stated above, most flucytosine use is in combination with an amphotericin B formulation for treatment of cryptococcal meningitis. This combination may also be used to treat other forms of cryptococcal infection and, uncommonly, to treat *Candida* infection. It may be an acceptable option for the clearance of candiduria in patients who cannot receive fluconazole because of allergy or resistance, but the number of patients who require this therapy is small.

Don't Forget!

Follow your patient's cell counts closely and consider dose modification or discontinuation if hematologic toxicity develops.

31

Azoles

Introduction to Azoles

Agents: ketoconazole, fluconazole,
itraconazole, voriconazole, posaconazole,
isavuconazole, multiple topical formulations

The azoles are a broad class of antifungal agents
whose drug development has recently been expand-
ing. They work by inhibiting fungal cytochrome
P450, decreasing ergosterol production. One might
expect that this mechanism of action would lead to
issues with drug interactions, and this is indeed a
significant problem with these drugs. While most
drug interactions can be successfully dealt with by
dosage adjustment, this is not true for all of them.
Also, remember that any dose adjustments made
while a patient is receiving an interacting drug
need to be readjusted when the therapy with the
interactor is finished.

Azoles have become mainstays of antifungal
pharmacotherapy. As they have been developed,
agents of variable antifungal spectrums and toxicity profiles have been introduced. These differences
are fundamental and are among the most important characteristics to know if you use them clinically. Because they are so different, we discuss the
commonly used systemic agents individually.

Fluconazole

The introduction of fluconazole in 1990 was a breakthrough in antifungal pharmacotherapy. Fluconazole is highly bioavailable, available in both oral and IV formulations, and highly active against many species of *Candida*. Before this, clinicians were faced with the toxicity and inconvenience of amphotericin B for serious forms of candidiasis. Fluconazole has a low incidence of serious adverse reactions, and converting from IV to oral therapy is simple. Though a shift toward non-*albicans* species of *Candida* has affected the use of fluconazole, it remains an important, frequently utilized agent.

Mechanism of Action

All azoles inhibit fungal cytochrome P450 14-alpha demethylase, inhibiting the conversion of lanosterol into ergosterol, which is a component of the fungal cell membrane.

Spectrum

Good: Candida albicans, Candida tropicalis, Candida parapsilosis, Candida lusitaniae, Cryptococcus neoformans, Coccidioides immitis

Moderate: Candida glabrata (can be susceptible
   dose-dependent, or resistant)
Poor: molds, many dimorphic fungi, *Candida krusei*

Adverse Effects

Though fluconazole is generally well tolerated, it
can cause hepatotoxicity or rash. It has a lower
propensity for serious drug interaction than many
other azoles, but interactions still occur with many
drugs metabolized by the cytochrome P450 system.
QTc prolongation is also possible.

Dosing Issues

Fluconazole doses for systemic fungal infections
may be escalated, particularly for the treatment
of *Candida glabrata* infections. Be sure to adjust
dosing with regard to renal function, because the
drug is eliminated through the urine. Vulvovaginal
candidiasis requires only a one-time dose of 150 mg
of fluconazole.

Important Facts

- Fluconazole is poorly active against all *Candida krusei* and some *Candida glabrata*.
  If you are using it for the latter infection,
  it is best to check susceptibilities and give
  800 mg/day of fluconazole after a loading dose.
  If your lab does not do susceptibility testing of
  fungi, consider an alternative agent such as
  an echinocandin.
- Fluconazole is often given as prophylaxis
  against *Candida* infections in susceptible
  populations like intensive care unit patients
  or patients with some cancers. Are you

treating a patient who was receiving it and now has yeast in the blood? Try an echinocandin instead (since they may have fluconazole-resistant *Candida*).

* The high bioavailability of fluconazole makes it an excellent therapy to transition to as patients tolerate oral medications.

What It's Good For

Fluconazole remains a drug of choice for many susceptible fungal infections, including invasive and noninvasive candidiasis and cryptococcal disease. It is also used for some dimorphic fungal infections, such as coccidioidomycosis.

Don't Forget!

Not all species of *Candida* are fluconazole-susceptible. Ensure that you check your patient's isolate before committing to a definitive course of therapy with it.

Itraconazole

Itraconazole is a broader-spectrum azole than flu-conazole that could probably have a bigger place in antifungal pharmacotherapy today if it were not for pharmacokinetic issues that have hampered its greater use. It has activity against *Aspergillus* and other mold species and was once commonly used as a step-down therapy in aspergillosis, but this use has declined since voriconazole became available.

Mechanism of Action

All azoles inhibit fungal cytochrome P450 14-alpha demethylase, inhibiting the conversion of lanos-terol into ergosterol, which is a component of the fungal cell membrane.

Spectrum

Good: *Candida albicans, Candida tropicalis, Candida parapsilosis, Candida lusitaniae, Cryptococcus neoformans, Aspergillus* species, many dimorphic fungi

Moderate: *Candida glabrata, Candida krusei*

Poor: Mucorales, many other molds

Adverse Effects

Itraconazole's adverse effect profile causes more concerns than that of fluconazole. In addition to causing hepatotoxicity, itraconazole is a negative ionotrope and is contraindicated in patients with heart failure. The oral solution is associated with diarrhea. It is also a stronger inhibitor of cytochrome P450 enzymes and has a long list of drug interactions. QTc prolongation can also occur.

Important Facts

- Itraconazole comes in two different formulations with different bioavailabilities and requirements. The capsules have lower bioavailability than the solution and are less preferred for systemic fungal infections.
- The oral formulations of itraconazole have different instructions with regard to taking them with meals. Capsules should always be taken with a full meal, whereas the solution should be taken on an empty stomach. Absorption can also be lowered by agents that decrease gastric acidity, such as proton-pump inhibitors; try having your patients take their itraconazole with a soda.
- Because itraconazole absorption is so erratic and unpredictable, concentrations are often monitored. Consider checking a trough concentration on your patient if he or she is taking it for a serious fungal infection and/or for a long time.
- Itraconazole was once available in an IV formulation, but this has been discontinued by the manufacturer. Ignore older references that suggest using it.

What It's Good For

Itraconazole remains a drug of choice for some dimorphic fungal infections, like histoplasmosis. It once had a larger role in the management and prophylaxis of aspergillosis and other mold infections, but it has been largely replaced by voriconazole. Itraconazole capsules are also used for the treatment of onychomycosis.

Don't Forget!

Watch for those drug interactions, and be sure to counsel your patients on how to take their itraconazole formulation.

Voriconazole

The introduction of voriconazole represented a significant improvement in the treatment of mold infections. It is also a broad-spectrum antifungal like itraconazole, with good activity against *Candida* species and many molds. Unlike itraconazole, voriconazole is well absorbed and available in both highly bioavailable oral formulations and an IV admixture. Most importantly, voriconazole was shown to be superior to amphotericin B deoxycholate for invasive aspergillosis and has become the drug of choice for that disease. With widespread use, however, limitations in terms of highly variable pharmacokinetics and long-term adverse effects have emerged.

Mechanism of Action

All azoles inhibit fungal cytochrome P450 14-alpha demethylase, inhibiting the conversion of lanosterol into ergosterol, which is a component of the fungal cell membrane.

Spectrum

Good: *Candida albicans, Candida lusitaniae, Candida parapsilosis, Candida tropicalis, Candida krusei, Cryptococcus neoformans, Aspergillus* species, many other molds

Moderate: Candida glabrata, Candida albicans that are fluconazole-resistant, *Fusarium* species
Poor: Mucorales

Adverse Effects

In addition to the hepatotoxicity, rash, and drug interactions that are common with this class, voriconazole has some agent-specific adverse effects worth watching.

Renal: The cyclodextrin solubilizer that intravenous voriconazole comes in is known to accumulate in renal dysfunction. This vehicle is thought to be nephrotoxic, but it is almost certainly less nephrotoxic that amphotericin B, so the use of intravenous voriconazole with renally insufficient patients is a risk/reward equation that should be considered with each patient.

Visual effects: Visual effects such as seeing wavy lines or halos around bright lights are very common and dose-related; they tend to go away with continued use.

Central nervous system effects: Distinct from the common visual effects of voriconazole, patients sometimes experience visual and auditory hallucinations. These effects are not permanent and tend to occur at higher voriconazole levels (especially during peak concentration periods).

Dermatologic: Voriconazole has long been known to cause sun sensitivity and patients should be advised to use sunscreen and avoid excessive sun exposure. Because voriconazole has been shown to be so useful for treating and preventing fungal infections, it has been used for durations far exceeding those studied in clinical trials. However, some studies now suggest an association between prolonged voriconazole use and certain skin cancers. Thus, it is even more essential to counsel patients on reducing sun exposure if they are taking voriconazole

Dosing Issues

Voriconazole has highly variable interpatient pharmacokinetics and nonlinear elimination, making it difficult to dose correctly. If you are committing your patient to an extended course of therapy for voriconazole, the standard of care has become to monitor serum drug concentrations (usually a trough level). There is no official consensus, but trough concentrations in the range of 2–5 mg/L are usually considered to be in the therapeutic window.

Important Facts

- Voriconazole is active against some fluconazole-resistant strains of *Candida albicans*, but it is less active against them than fluconazole-susceptible strains. An echinocandin is a better choice, but consider susceptibility testing if you need to use voriconazole for an oral option.
- Voriconazole is a potent inhibitor and a substrate of the cytochrome P450 system. The list of drugs that interact with voriconazole is long and varied. Some of them are contraindicated, such as rifampin, while others, such as calcineurin inhibitors (e.g., cyclosporine) require dose adjustments. This is significant because many of the patients who require voriconazole are immunosuppressed.

- The IV form of voriconazole contains a cyclo-dextrin vehicle that accumulates in renal dysfunction and may be nephrotoxic. It is contraindicated with a creatinine clearance of less than 50 ml/min. The oral formulations avoid this issue.
- Voriconazole is eliminated hepatically and is unlikely to be useful in the treatment of candiduria.

What It's Good For

Voriconazole is a drug of choice for invasive aspergillosis and is frequently used in the treatment of infections caused by other molds. It can be used for candidiasis as well, but fluconazole and echinocandins are more frequently used for these infections. Some clinicians use voriconazole in the empiric treatment of febrile neutropenia.

Don't Forget!

Watch for drug interactions with voriconazole, and consider checking drug concentrations if you are using it for an extended course of therapy.

Posaconazole

Posaconazole is an analog of itraconazole that is substantially more active against many fungi. Currently, it is indicated only for the prophylaxis of fungal infections patients and the treatment of oropharyngeal candidiasis. It was the first azole with good activity against Mucorales, a difficult-to-treat order of molds that most antifungals (voriconazole included) do not treat; however, the recently approved isavuconazole also has activity against these pathogens (see next section).

Mechanism of Action

All azoles inhibit fungal cytochrome P450 14-alpha demethylase, inhibiting the conversion of lanosterol into ergosterol, which is a component of the fungal cell membrane.

Spectrum

Good: *Candida albicans, Candida lusitaniae, Candida parapsilosis, Candida tropicalis, Candida krusei, Aspergillus* species, Mucorales, many other molds, dimorphic fungi
Moderate: *Fusarium* species, *Candida glabrata*

Though posaconazole is active against these organisms, comparative clinical trial data are lacking for many of them.

Adverse Reactions

Posaconazole seems to be well tolerated, though it can cause hepatotoxicity, nausea, and rash. It has a similar propensity to cause drug interactions via cytochrome P450 as the other azoles.

Dosing Issues

A key limitation to posaconazole's use was its initial availability only as an oral suspension. This formulation requires administration with food to increase its absorption; foods with a high fat concentration, nutritional supplements containing fat, and low-pH beverages like soda all increase absorption. Even under the best circumstances, absorption of the suspension is limited and variable. Recently a delayed-release tablet formulation has been approved that achieves much higher and more reliable concentrations. Note, however, that the tablet cannot be crushed or chewed. There is also an IV formulation.

▓ Important Facts

- Posaconazole's most common use has been in the prophylaxis of fungal infections in high-risk patients. As with voriconazole, many of these patients are taking immunosuppressants that interact with posaconazole, so keep close tabs on those drug concentrations.
- The *in vitro* activity of posaconazole against *Aspergillus* is generally similar to that of voriconazole, but the lack of clinical trial data comparing posaconazole to voriconazole (or even to amphotericin) for this infection has made many clinicians hesitant to use it as a first-line

agent, even though it is better tolerated than voriconazole.

- As noted, posaconazole oral suspension has issues with absorption. High-fat meals and acidic beverages boost absorption substantially and may be required for adequate absorption in some patients. Proton-pump inhibitors lower absorption and administering with a soda is not enough to overcome this factor. Posaconazole drug concentrations are available and should probably be considered for patients with questionable absorption, or if posaconazole is being used for treatment of invasive infections.

What It's Good For

Posaconazole is most commonly used as prophylaxis against fungal infections in susceptible hosts, but it can also be used in mucormycosis, oropharyngeal candidiasis, and fungal infections refractory to other agents. As noted earlier, a limitation to its more widespread use is a lack of clinical trial data.

Don't Forget!

As with itraconazole, it is vitally important to know which oral formulation—capsules or suspension—your patient is taking. Dosing and administration are very different between the two.

Isavuconazole

The newest azole antifungal is isavuconazole. In many ways isavuconazole is similar to what posaconazole now offers. It has an expanded spectrum of activity that includes *Candida*, *Aspergillus*, and Mucorales. It is available as IV and oral formulations, has P450-mediated drug interactions, and a toxicity profile that is most concerning for hepatic effects. A key difference is that isavuconazole's FDA approval was based on clinical trials in invasive aspergillosis and mucormycosis—two areas where posaconazole currently lacks clinical trial data. However, posaconazole has more extensive clinical use.

Mechanism of Action

All azoles inhibit fungal cytochrome P450 14-alpha demethylase, inhibiting the conversion of lanosterol into ergosterol, which is a component of the fungal cell membrane.

Spectrum

Good: *Candida* spp (see later, the section "Important Facts" regarding clinical trial data about isavuconazole in invasive candidiasis), *Aspergillus* species, Mucorales, some other molds and dimorphic fungi

Moderate: Candida glabrata
Poor: Fusarium species

Adverse Reactions

Based on clinical trial data, hepatotoxicity on a similar level to other azole antifungals is anticipated (although it may be somewhat less frequent than with voriconazole). Interestingly, unlike other azoles isavuconazole does not appear to prolong the QT interval but can actually shorten it. This does not seem to have clinical significance besides among patients with congenitally short QT intervals, and may allow for use of isavuconazole in patients with prolonged QT intervals who would be at risk of an arrhythmia if prescribed a different azole antifungal.

Dosing Issues

The bioavailability of isavuconazole's oral formulation (a capsule) is excellent and not affected by food or gastric acidity. However, the capsules are hard and not designed to be opened, crushed, or chewed which limits their administration among patients with feeding tubes or swallowing issues. Isavuconazole has a very long half-life and so to attain therapeutic levels more rapidly, there is an extensive loading dose regimen: administration every 8 hours for six doses (48 hours), before transition to a once-daily maintenance regimen. Isavuconazole is supplied as a prodrug (isavucazonium sulfate) that is hydrolysed to isavuconazole after administration; however, this makes for funky dosing: 372 mg of isavucazonium yields 200 mg of isavuconazole. This leads to the potential for confusion in ordering doses.

Important Facts

- Isavuconazole has *in vitro* activity against *Candida* species similar to that of voriconazole and posaconazole. A phase III randomized clinical trial was performed against caspofungin among patients with invasive *Candida* infections. The conclusion of this study was that isavuconazole was not noninferior to caspofungin in the treatment of these infections—the FDA is not going to be granting isavuconazole an indication for invasive candidiasis any time soon. However, whether or not isavuconazole is a worse option than voriconazole or posaconazole for these infections is a matter of debate. Posaconazole has FDA approval for only the less-severe oropharyngeal candidiasis and has not been studied in clinical trials for invasive candidiasis. Voriconazole is FDA approved for invasive candidiasis based on the results of a study comparing it to conventional amphotericin B followed by fluconazole. Subsequent studies have suggested that echinocandins may be more effective than both amphotericin and fluconazole in treatment of invasive *Candida* infections. Thus, isavuconazole may have suffered the misfortune of being compared against the most effective anti-*Candida* agent (echinocandins) while voriconazole got to "play against the JV team" and posaconazole was not even studied. The bottom line: for invasive candidiasis, whenever possible use an echinocandin (most effective) or fluconazole (balance of efficacy and convenience).

- Isavuconazole's pharmacokinetics is more predictable than voriconazole's and possibly posaconazole's; however, clinicians are frequently reassured by demonstrating adequate serum drug levels. Currently, fewer laboratories offer isavuconazole levels than voriconazole or posaconazole levels, but this is likely to increase over time.

What It's Good For

There is not extensive experience with isavuconazole yet, but based on its trial data it appears to be a good option for invasive mold infections.

Don't Forget!

Double-check that dosing—it's important to give the correct dose as well as the full loading regimen; otherwise your patient will take a week to get to a subtherapeutic steady-state.

32

Echinocandins

The echinocandins are the latest class of antifungal agents to be introduced in clinical practice and have changed the way some fungal diseases are treated. Their mechanism of action is distinct from that of other antifungals and gives clinicians a new area of fungi to target. The three available echinocandins are similar drugs with virtually indistinguishable spectra. They are very well tolerated and have excellent activity against *Candida*, but they all suffer from the same pharmacokinetic setback: lack of an oral formulation. They have considerably fewer drug interactions than azoles, are safer than polyenes, and have great activity against fluconazole-resistant yeasts.

Mechanism of Action

Echinocandins inhibit beta-1,3-D-glucan synthase, the enzyme responsible for the production of beta-1,3-D-glucan, a vital component of the cell wall of many fungi. They are only active against fungi that are dependent this type of glucan.

Spectrum

Good: Candida albicans, Candida glabrata, Candida lusitaniae, Candida parapsilosis, Candida tropicalis, Candida krusei, Aspergillus species

Moderate: Candida parapsilosis, some dimorphic fungi, Mucorales (in combination with amphotericin B)

Poor: most non-Aspergillus molds, Cryptococcus neoformans

Adverse Effects

Echinocandins have an excellent safety profile. They can cause mild histamine-mediated infusion-related reactions, but these are not common and can be ameliorated by slowing the infusion rate. Hepatotoxicity is also possible with any of these agents, but this is not common.

Important Facts

- Differences among the echinocandins are minor and mostly pharmacokinetic. Caspofungin and micafungin are eliminated hepatically by noncytochrome P450 metabolism, while anidulafungin degrades in the plasma and avoids hepatic metabolism. Despite this unique method of elimination, it is not completely devoid of hepatotoxicity.

- Echinocandins have excellent fungicidal activity against *Candida*, but against *Aspergillus* species they exhibit activity that is neither classically cidal nor static. Instead, they cause aberrant, nonfunctional hyphae to be formed by the actively growing mold.

- The echinocandins are only modestly active against molds, but do appear to substantially enhance the effects of other antifungals against these pathogens. A randomized controlled trial of voriconazole with or without anidulafungin in invasive aspergillosis showed a trend toward reduced mortality among patients receiving combination therapy (the difference was not statistically significant—$p = 0.07$—but given the low toxicity of echinocandins many clinicians refuse to submit to the tyranny of the p-value and advocate for the use of this combination therapy). The echinocandins may also enhance the efficacy of liposomal amphotericin B against Mucorales infections, based on *in vitro* and limited clinical data.
- Though drug interactions with the echinocandins are minor, you should be aware of some of them, particularly with caspofungin and micafungin. Be careful when you use them with the immunosuppressants cyclosporine (caspofungin) and sirolimus (micafungin).

What They're Good For

Echinocandins are drugs of choice for invasive candidiasis, particularly in patients who are clinically unstable or if there is a risk the infection is caused by an azole-resistant species. They are also useful in the treatment of invasive aspergillosis but do not have the level of supporting data that voriconazole and the polyenes do for this indication. All of them are used for esophageal candidiasis, and some are used in prophylaxis or empiric therapy of fungal infections in neutropenic patients. Some clinicians will add an echinocandin to voriconazole (for *Aspergillus* infections) or an amphotericin B formulation (versus Mucorales) in an attempt to increase likelihood of cure for these infections.

Don't Forget!

Echinocandins are great drugs for invasive candidiasis, but they are not cheap and IV therapy can be inconvenient. After beginning empiric therapy with an echinocandin, consider transitioning your patient to fluconazole if he or she has a susceptible strain of *Candida* and no contraindication to fluconazole.

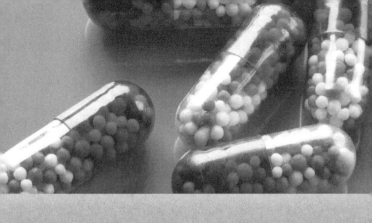

Antiviral Drugs

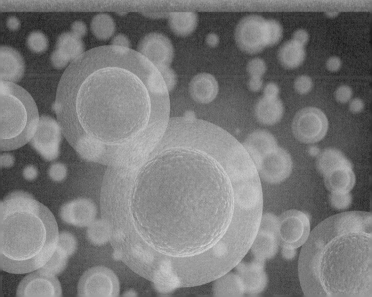

PART 5

Antiviral Drugs

Introduction to Antiviral Drugs

The term *virus* has interesting meanings in popular culture: it is commonly used to describe something that has or can spread quickly from person to person, such as a computer virus or a "viral" video, a video that gains quick popularity through Internet or e-mail sharing. This usage represents a basic understanding of the high transmissibility of many respiratory viruses, such as influenza and the rhinoviruses that cause the common cold. However, many less-understood viruses, particularly those that cause chronic disease, can be confusing.

The world of viruses is very different from that of prokaryotes and eukaryotes. Viruses are dependent on cells to replicate and cannot perpetuate without them. They are considerably smaller than eukaryotes and even much smaller than most prokaryotes, though they vary widely in size (see Figure 1–2). They are relatively simple organisms compared with prokaryotes or eukaryotes, but they outnumber all other life forms on earth. Scientists have debated for many years about whether viruses are life forms or not, and no clear consensus yet exists. The understanding of how they interact with and shape the existence of living cells, however, has increased greatly since they were described by Louis Pasteur in the late nineteenth century.

An in-depth discussion of the structure of viruses is beyond the scope of this text, but a basic understanding of viruses will help you understand the actions of antiviral drugs. Viruses are highly diverse, though nearly all of them share a few common characteristics. Many are covered by a viral *envelope* as their outmost layer, composed of elements of the host cell membrane, endoplasmic reticulum, or nuclear envelope. This layer covers the *capsid*, a shell composed of identical building blocks of *capsomeres*. The capsid protects the viral *nucleic acid*, which is either DNA or RNA but not both (as in cells). The DNA or RNA can be either single- or double-stranded. Finally, many viruses contain enzymes that catalyze reactions that lead to their replication or cell entry. Viruses cannot synthesize their own components to replicate— they are dependent on host cellular processes for all synthetic functions. Individual complete particles of virus are termed *virions*.

The specific steps of the viral life cycle differ from virus to virus, but they follow the same basic pathway. Viruses spread from host to host through various means, some through direct inhalation, some through direct fluid exchange, some through vectors such as mosquitoes. Once a virus reaches its target cell, it has to penetrate the cell membrane. Specific receptors on the cell and viral surfaces often facilitate this process. The virus then uncoats and releases its genetic information from the capsule into the host cell. The host cell reads the genetic material and begins to translate it into viral proteins. How exactly this proceeds depends on the form in which the genetic material exists in the virus. In some cases, the genetic material is encoded as RNA. For some RNA viruses, host cell ribosomes translate the RNA into proteins. In the group of viruses known as retroviruses, the RNA genetic material is first translated into DNA (via an enzyme known as reverse transcriptase) before integrating into the host genome. For these viruses or those viruses whose genome is already encoded as DNA, transcription into messenger RNA occurs, followed by translation into protein. Once the pieces of the puzzle are built, the viral enzymes assemble them into complete virions and they are finally released from the cell. The available antiviral drugs are aimed at various steps in this cycle. Some are aimed at specific receptors against specific viruses (such as influenza), and some are aimed at more general steps to attack multiple viruses.

The pharmacotherapy of viral infections is different from that of bacterial infections. Patient-specific susceptibility results are rarely available, leaving practitioners to choose therapies based upon general patterns of susceptibility for that type of virus (HIV is a notable exception, where susceptibility testing is a standard of care). While viruses can be cultured, many viral illnesses are diagnosed through genetic testing for viral antigens or nucleic acids. These tests can be followed quantitatively to see if an infection improves, but symptoms are usually followed instead. Most common viral infections have no effective pharmacotherapeutic remedy, which is a fancy way of saying that there is still "no cure for the common cold."

Agents: acyclovir, valacyclovir, famciclovir

These agents are primarily used in the treatment of infections caused by herpes simplex virus (HSV) and varicella-zoster virus (VZV), though they are active against some other viruses as well. Acyclovir is poorly absorbed and must be given up to five times daily when administered orally; valacyclovir and famciclovir are pro-drugs that are absorbed better and can be administered less frequently. Only acyclovir can be administered intravenously, and it is the agent of choice for serious HSV infections such as encephalitis.

Mechanism of Action

These drugs are nucleoside analogs that, after phosphorylation, are incorporated into the elongating viral DNA strand just like cellular nucleotides; but they lack the functional group that allows the next nucleotide to be added, halting replication.

Spectrum

Good: HSV-1 and HSV-2
Moderate: VZV
Poor: Epstein-Barr virus (EBV), cytomegalovirus (CMV), HIV

Adverse Effects

These drugs are generally well tolerated with few adverse effects. The most concerning adverse effect is nephrotoxicity through either crystallization or acute interstitial nephritis (AIN), most commonly associated with IV acyclovir in higher doses. Crystallization is preventable through hydration and correct dosing in renally impaired patients. Seizures, tremors, or other CNS effects can also occur. Nausea, diarrhea, and rash are more common. Thrombotic thrombocytopenic purpura has been reported with valacyclovir in HIV patients.

Important Facts

- Valacyclovir is a pro-drug of acyclovir with substantially improved bioavailability and less-frequent dosing. Its disadvantage is higher cost. Famciclovir is a pro-drug of penciclovir, an agent that is available only as a topical preparation.
- Acyclovir dosing varies widely by indication and host status. Be sure to double-check that it is appropriate for your patients.
- Acyclovir is most nephrotoxic in combination with diuretics or other nephrotoxins. Keep your patients hydrated during acyclovir therapy, particularly if it is given in higher IV doses.

What They're Good For

Acyclovir is the drug of choice for severe or difficult-to-treat HSV infections, such as encephalitis or severe HSV outbreaks among HIV patients. Any of these agents can be used to treat HSV-2 infections (genital herpes) to prevent outbreaks or decrease symptom duration. They are all also effective in treating VZV infection.

Don't Forget!

Make sure your patient can afford valacyclovir or famciclovir before prescribing either one. Oral acyclovir is less convenient, but much less expensive.

Anti-cytomegalovirus Agents

35

Cytomegalovirus (CMV) causes infections that are usually asymptomatic in immunocompetent patients but can be devastating in immunocompromised patients. Approximately 60% of Americans become seropositive for CMV by adulthood, and infection is lifelong. If a patient becomes immunocompromised, the infection can reactivate and the patient will need pharmacotherapy. Anticytomegalovirus agents work by preventing viral replication. They also all have appreciable toxicity that must be respected and monitored.

Mechanisms of Action

Ganciclovir is a nucleoside analogue that, after phosphorylation, is integrated into viral DNA by DNA polymerase, halting viral replication. Valganciclovir is a pro-drug of ganciclovir. Cidofovir is a nucleotide analogue that has a similar mechanism to ganciclovir.

Foscarnet is a pyrophosphate analogue that acts as a noncompetitive inhibitor of the DNA and RNA polymerases of multiple viruses.

Good: CMV, HSV-1, HSV-2, VZV, EBV
Poor: HIV

Ganciclovir and valganciclovir are the same active drug and have the same adverse reactions. They both have dose-dependent myelosuppression that is relatively common, particularly when used in higher doses or in renally impaired patients without dose adjustment. Foscarnet is nephrotoxic and neurotoxic, and it is reserved for patients who have failed other therapy. Nausea, vomiting, and diarrhea can occur from any of these agents. Foscarnet can also cause penile ulcers. Cidofovir is an uncommonly used agent that also exhibits nephrotoxicity.

Important Facts

- Oral ganciclovir has been replaced by valganciclovir, which has much better bioavailability.
- Ganciclovir must be carefully dosed by patient weight and renal function. Monitor patients closely for changes in renal function when they are on therapy.
- The package insert for valganciclovir specifies dose adjustment for renal dysfunction but not weight. It comes in two strengths: 900 mg and 450 mg. The dose of 900 mg BID is considered to be equivalent to 5 mg/kg q12h of IV ganciclovir, but it may be much more than that for an underweight patient because it is

approximately 60% bioavailable. Consider this example for a 50-kg patient:

Ganciclovir dose = 50 kg × 5 mg/kg = 250 mg ganciclovir

Valganciclovir dose = 900 mg × 0.60 bioavailability = 540 mg of active ganciclovir

This patient would receive more than double the amount of active ganciclovir if 900 mg BID of valganciclovir were used. It thus may be worth considering dose reduction in underweight patients, particularly if they are at high risk of toxicity.

- The nephrotoxicity of foscarnet and cidofovir is such that both require extensive prehydration regimens with normal saline to reduce the toxicity risk. Cidofovir actually requires coadministration with probenecid, which reduces the excretion of cidofovir into the renal tubules and attenuates its toxicity.
- It takes awhile, but genotype-based susceptibility testing is available for CMV and is usually performed if resistance is suspected in patients not responding to ganciclovir. The genotype will reveal whether ganciclovir resistance is present and whether cidofovir or foscarnet are therapeutic options.

What They're Good For

Ganciclovir and valganciclovir are first-line drugs for the treatment and prevention of CMV infections. Valganciclovir is often given to prevent CMV infection after transplant. Foscarnet is a second-line agent for CMV that can also be used for severe or resistant HSV infections. Cidofovir is a second-line agent for CMV.

Don't Forget!

Although valganciclovir is oral, it is has good bioavailabity and has adverse effects identical to those of ganciclovir. Valganciclovir use requires monitoring for toxicity that is just as rigorous as that for intravenous ganciclovir.

Neuraminidase Inhibitors

36

The neuraminidase inhibitors are anti-influenza virus drugs that have activity against influenza A and B strains, unlike amandatine and rimantidine, older drugs that are active only against influenza A strains. They work by preventing the viral neuraminidase enzyme from releasing new virions from the host cell, preventing further replication. The three drugs differ in their forms of delivery: oseltamivir is an oral pro-drug, while peramivir is intravenous, and zanamivir is inhaled. They can be used in either the treatment of influenza or as prophylaxis for patients who cannot take the influenza vaccine.

Mechanism of Action

These drugs are competitive inhibitors of viral neuraminidase, an enzyme responsible for several functions of the influenza virus, including the release of new virions from infected cells.

Spectrum

Good: influenza A and B
Poor: other viruses

Adverse Effects

All three agents are generally well tolerated. Oseltamivir can cause nausea, vomiting, and abdominal pain, but these tend to be transient effects. Headache and fatigue can also occur, particularly during prophylactic use when the drug is given for a longer period of time. Zanamivir has mostly pulmonary adverse effects, including cough and bronchospasm. Avoid using it in patients with asthma or other reactive pulmonary diseases. Peramivir doesn't seem to have any characteristic adverse effects based on limited experience to date.

Important Facts

- Neuraminidase inhibitors are most effective when started early in the course of infection, because viral replication peaks early (48–72 hours after infection). The package inserts for these drugs state they should be started in patients who have been symptomatic for no more than 2 days—this is based on the labeled indications for mild–moderate infection in healthy adults. In severe influenza infections such as those that require hospitalization or in vulnerable patients, data suggest there may be benefit even if therapy is delayed and so treatment guidelines recommend initiating treatment even if outside the "window" for these patients.
- Resistance to the neuraminidase inhibitors can occur. Their utility is dictated by the degree of resistance that exists in the dominant influenza strains of the season. Currently, zanamivir is active against the vast majority of oseltamivir- and peramivir-resistant strains, but these resistance patterns may change.

- Oseltamivir and zanamivir are highly effective at preventing influenza infection when the predominant strains in the community are susceptible, but they are not substitutes for a vaccination strategy. Adverse effects are more common with the prolonged use seen with prophylactic use than with the shorter durations of therapeutic use.

What They're Good For

All three agents are effective at treating and preventing influenza infections if the circulating strains are susceptible—although the vast majority of data was among patients with "uncomplicated" influenza (despite the fact that the complicated patients are those who are most in need of effective therapy). The desired route of administration dictates the choice of agent.

Don't Forget!

If your patient is otherwise healthy and their flu has peaked and he or she is improving, then it's probably not the time to start one of these drugs. It may, however, be a great time to counsel on the utility of the influenza vaccine for next season.

Antiretroviral Drugs

37

Introduction to Antiretroviral Drugs

Despite the decades-long stall in antimicrobial drug development, one area that has seen substantial growth is the development of antiretroviral drugs targeting the HIV virus. Only a single active drug (zidovudine) was available near the beginning of the epidemic in the mid-1980s, and today more than two dozen drugs and drug combinations are available with more in the pipeline. Some antiretroviral drug classes are in their second or third generation of agents, leaving some of the earlier agents essentially obsolete. The development and proper usage of these agents have moved HIV infection toward the realm of a chronic disease rather than a short-term "death sentence." More than any other antimicrobial group, however, the antiretrovirals come with the challenges of taking complex multidrug regimens for years: drug adherence, resistance, toxicities, and interactions. The full scope of these issues is beyond this text; instead, we will highlight key aspects of the drug classes and unique properties of individual agents, especially as related to toxicities. The treatment recommendations for HIV change at a dizzying pace; when determining whether a patient's regimen meets the most updated guidelines, we recommend you check the Website at http://aidsinfo.nih.gov. *Important note:* We present the commonly used abbreviations for these agents so that you may recognize them in practice, but it is not acceptable to use these abbreviations in prescriptions and it is not recommended to use them in patient documentation.

Nucleoside and Nucleotide Reverse Transcriptase Inhibitors

Agents: tenofovir disoproxil fumarate (TDF), tenofovir alafenamide (TAF), emtricitabine (FTC), lamivudine (3TC), abacavir (ABC), zidovudine (ZDV, AZT), stavudine (d4T), didanosine (ddI)

Combinations: emtricitabine/tenofovir disoproxil fumarate (Truvada), abacavir/lamivudine (Epzicom), emtricitabine/tenofovir alafenamide (Descovy), lamivudine/zidovudine (Combivir), abacavir/lamivudine/zidovudine (Trizivir)

The nucleoside reverse transcriptase inhibitors (NRTIs) are the oldest class of antiretrovirals (tenofovir is technically a nucleotide but is grouped with these agents). A combination of two of these drugs typically forms the "backbone" of most anti-HIV regimens.

Mechanism of Action

The NRTIs inhibit the action of the virally encoded protein reverse transcriptase by taking the place of nucleotides in the elongating strand of viral DNA, leading to early termination of the viral DNA strain.

Spectrum

In addition to being used to treat the HIV virus, several of these drugs (tenofovir, emtricitabine, lamivudine) have clinically useful activity against hepatitis B virus (HBV).

Adverse Effects

Note that some of the more problematic agents from a toxicity perspective (didanosine, stavudine, zidovudine) are used uncommonly in current treatment regimens.

Extremities: Peripheral neuropathy is seen as a delayed, slowly progressive adverse effect in some patients taking didanosine or stavudine (and especially in combination).

Gastrointestinal: NRTIs tend to have less GI toxicity (nausea, vomiting, diarrhea) than many antiretrovirals, but zidovudine and didanosine may be problematic.

Hematologic: Bone marrow suppression (anemia, neutropenia) occurs frequently with zidovudine, and rarely with other NRTIs.

Hypersensitivity: In a minority of patients, abacavir use is associated with a hypersensitivity reaction manifesting with fever, rash, and flulike symptoms days to weeks after starting therapy. Continuation of or rechallenge with abacavir in patients experiencing this syndrome can be fatal. Presence of the HLA-B*:5701 allele is predictive of toxicity, and routine screening of patients for this genotype is now recommended before starting therapy; patients testing positive should not be offered abacavir.

Metabolic: Lactic acidosis, hepatic steatosis, and pancreatitis are part of a complex of toxicities suspected to be of mitochondrial origin that are a classwide adverse effect of NRTIs. Mortality can be high if symptoms are not recognized early—which is a problem because symptoms are typically delayed (for months) in onset and may be nonspecific in initial presentation. Agents with a higher propensity for this toxicity include stavudine, didanosine, and zidovudine. Didanosine and zidovudine may also contribute to hyperlipidemia, insulin resistance, and lipoatrophy (loss of fat causing changes in appearance, primarily in the face and buttocks).

Renal: Nephrotoxicity, evidenced by increased serum creatinine and renal electrolyte and protein wasting, is a well-documented adverse effect of tenofovir and requires regular monitoring of renal function. The new formulation tenofovir alafenamide (TAF) appears to confer less toxicity risk than the tenofovir disoporoxil fumarate (TDF) formulation—however, TDF use alone or in combination pills is very widespread and it may be a long time before TAF replaces TDF.

Important Facts

- Most of the NRTIs require dosage adjustment in renal dysfunction. This may require avoiding the fixed-dose combination preparations to give more dose flexibility.
- NRTIs have fewer metabolic drug interactions compared with the other antiretroviral drug

classes. Tenofovir should not be coadministred with didanosine and when given with atazanavir may require dosage adjustment of atazanavir.

- Various patterns of cross-resistance among the NRTIs occur. Expert interpretation of antiviral susceptibility is required, and in some cases NRTIs may confer a therapeutic benefit even for resistant viruses.
- The new tenofovir formulation (TAF) has a much lower dose than the TDF version. Careful attention to which formulation is planned to be used is important to avoid medication errors.

What They're Good For

NRTIs are used as components of a combination antiretroviral regimen for HIV. For treatment-naïve patients, two NRTIs are typically combined with a drug from another class. For treatment-experienced patients, three or more NRTIs may be part of a salvage regimen. As noted, certain NRTIs are also used to manage HBV infections. Use of these drugs in management of HIV/HBV coinfected patients requires accounting for the overlap in activity between the viruses to ensure that resistance doesn't emerge because of suboptimal activity against one of the viruses.

Don't Forget!

If there aren't two NRTIs (taking into account combination preparations as well) as part of a patient's anti-HIV regimen, something is weird. The patient may be on an unusual salvage regimen (hopefully under the care of an HIV expert), but it's best to check to make sure something didn't get left out.

Non-nucleoside Reverse Transcriptase Inhibitors (NNRTIs)

The non-nucleoside reverse transcriptase inhibitors (NNRTIs) inhibit the same enzyme as the NRTIs but work through a different mechanism and have greatly different pharmacologic properties. That extra N makes a big difference: it's very important to keep the two drug classes straight.

Mechanism of Action

Instead of inhibiting the action of reverse transcriptase by "pretending" to be regular nucleosides, NNRTIs bind to a different part of the enzyme. The binding of the NNRTI causes a change in the conformation of the enzyme that interferes with its ability to form the viral DNA chain.

Spectrum

Only current clinical use is for HIV.

Adverse Effects

CNS: Efavirenz can cause a broad spectrum of CNS effects; common effects include dizziness, drowsiness (or sometimes insomnia), and abnormal (and especially vivid) dreams. Less common effects include depression, psychosis, and suicidal ideation. The onset of effects is usually very rapid (with the first few doses) and often subsides after several weeks of therapy. These effects may be minimized by taking the drug on an empty stomach and by taking at bedtime or 2–3 hours prior. A history of mental illness or depression is a relative contraindication to the use of efavirenz.

Dermatologic: Rashes can occur with all NNRTIs, although nevirapine appears to be the biggest offender. Though some mild forms can be treated with antihistamines, any lesions involving the mucous membranes (suggesting Stevens-Johnson syndrome or similar eruptions) must be managed urgently and represent an absolute contraindication to rechallenge.

Hepatotoxicity: All NNRTIs can cause a spectrum of hepatotoxicity, from asymptomatic transaminase elevations, to clinical hepatitis, to fulminant hepatic failure. Nevirapine-induced hepatotoxicity may occur in the context of a hypersensitivity reaction (see next). Monitoring of signs and symptoms of hepatitis and liver enzymes is important for all these agents.

Hypersensitivity: Nevirapine can cause a hypersensitivity reaction characterized by flulike symptoms, fever, jaundice, and abdominal pain, with or without a rash. Fulminant hepatic failure and severe rash (e.g., toxic epidermal necrolysis) are the most feared manifestations of nevirapine hypersensitivity reactions. Interestingly, this syndrome appears to be more frequent in patients who are less immunocompromised (have higher CD4 counts) when starting nevirapine. The risk of nevirapine hypersensitivity syndrome may be reduced by using a "reverse taper" upon drug initiation: start with a lower dose and escalate to full dose over 2 weeks, when the risk is highest.

Metabolic: Lipohypertrophy, manifesting as a gradual accumulation of fat in the abdomen, chest, and neck (as a "buffalo hump"), may occur with the NNRTIs. Efavirenz and nevirapine have also been linked to hyperlipidemia. Compared to efavirenz, rilpivirine showed less of an effect on lipid profiles.

Pregnancy/Lactation: Efavirenz is a pregnancy category D agent and should not be offered to pregnant women or those trying to conceive or not using effective birth control. Other NNRTIs are pregnancy category C, except rilpivirine, which is category B.

Important Facts

- A key limitation of NNRTIs has been the low "genetic barrier" to resistance. A single point mutation can lead to high-level resistance to the entire class of drugs. Thus, even stricter adherence may be necessary to NNRTI-based regimens to prevent the emergence of resistance. The advanced-generation agents etravirine and rilpivirine possess activity against viruses with some NNRTI mutations and may have roles for patients who have failed either efavirenz or nevirapine.

- NNRTIs have a much broader drug interaction profile than the NRTIs (remember, one N makes a lot of difference!). Generally, nevirapine is an inducer of drug metabolism, efavirenz and etravirine show mixed inducing and inhibitory properties, and rilpivirine does not as yet appear to have significant effects on metabolism of other drugs. Concentrations of the NNRTIs can themselves be affected by inhibitors or inducers of drug-metabolizing enzymes. Thus, careful screening of these drugs against all other agents in a patient's regimen is warranted.

What They're Good For

A combination regimen of efavirenz with the NRTIs tenofovir and emtricitabine is one of the recommended alternative regimens for initial treatment of treatment-naïve patients with HIV. Co-formulated as Atripla, this regimen briefly held the title of the only one-pill, once-daily antiretroviral regimen and was a preferred initial regimen. New integrase strand transfer agents also offer this option now, with a lesser degree of toxicity and possibly a lower genetic barrier to resistance. The other NNRTIs tend to be used as second-line therapy in treatment-experienced patients.

Don't Forget!

When initiating an NNRTI, the first few weeks are key. Patients must be counseled carefully about recognizing adverse effects, especially skin reactions and symptoms of hepatotoxicity. The need for strict adherence to prevent resistance, the dose titration schedule for nevirapine, and the CNS effects of efavirenz must be fully explained to patients. There's really only one shot to get it right!

Protease Inhibitors

Agents: atazanavir (ATV), darunavir (DRV), ritonavir (boosting dose: /r), fosamprenavir (FPV), saquinavir (SQV), indinavir (IDV), nelfinavir (NFV), tipranavir (TPV), ritonavir (full dose: RTV)

Combinations: darunavir/cobicistat (DRV/c, Prezcobix), atazanavir/cobicistat (ATV/c, Evotaz), lopinavir/ritonavir (LPV/r, Kaletra)

The introduction of the protease inhibitors (PIs) was a major advance in antiretroviral therapy. Combination regimens with PIs were the beginning of the era of "highly active antiretroviral therapy" (HAART) and have had a major impact on prolonging lifespan among HIV-infected individuals. (*Note:* the term *HAART* has largely fallen out of favor.) PIs are now entering their third generation, with more-potent agents having fewer acute toxicities; however, long-term toxicities are arising as a concern. A key advance has been the introduction of "boosting": using the (normally undesirable) potent inhibition of drug-metabolizing enzymes displayed by the antiretroviral ritonavir or the pharmacokinetic booster cobicistat to increase the serum concentrations and half-lives of other PIs. Boosting is now routine for essentially all PIs: patients either take an additional pill of a low dose of ritonavir along with their PI (typically indicated as "/r", as in ATV/r) or a co-formulation with cobicistat ("/c", as in ATV/c) or ritonavir (as with LPV/r).

Mechanism of Action

When the hijacked HIV-infected cell uses the cell's ribosomes to synthesize its own proteins, some of them are created in long chains that need to be cut up into their component parts to work correctly. Protease inhibitors selectively inhibit the viral enzyme (HIV protease) responsible for this processing. Think of protease enzymes as a pair of scissors that cut out prefabricated shapes from a piece of cardboard paper—take away the scissors (with protease inhibitors) and the shapes are just a piece of paper.

Spectrum

Only current clinical use is for HIV. Protease inhibitors that treat hepatitis C virus (HCV) are different drugs and are not active against HIV, and vice versa.

Adverse Effects

Cardiovascular: Patients with HIV living long enough to suffer from heart attacks and strokes is viewed (somewhat perversely) as a sign of the success of potent antiretroviral therapy, particularly PIs. However, the possibility of cardiovascular adverse effects is now recognized as a substantial problem. PIs appear to interact with conventional cardiovascular risk factors to increase risk for myocardial infarction and stroke beyond that expected from just prolonging lifespan. Atazanavir and darunavir may confer somewhat lower risk compared with other PIs. Management is with all the mainstays of cardiovascular risk prevention (diet, exercise, drugs).

Gastrointestinal: All PIs are pretty hard on the GI tract (nausea, vomiting, diarrhea). Taking the drugs with food may reduce the symptoms somewhat. Many patients find the effects more tolerable with time. Severe cases may require administration with antiemetics or antidiarrheals.

Hepatotoxicity: The potential for hepatotoxicity exists with all PIs, ranging from asymptomatic transaminase elevations to clinical hepatitis. Risk may be highest with boosted tipranavir.

Metabolic: One means by which PIs increase cardiovascular risk is through adverse effects on the lipid profile. The PIs are also associated with lipodistrophy (fat accumulation in abdomen, breasts, and neck).

Nephrotoxicity: Renal toxicity caused by certain PIs precipitating in the kidneys or ureters has been reported. This toxicity is most common with the now infrequently used agent indinavir, and it is reported rarely with atazanavir and fosamprenavir. Adequate fluid intake is recommended for prevention.

Important Facts

- Compared with the NNRTIs and INSTIs, PIs are more robust to antiviral resistance. Typically, several mutations in the target enzyme are required to confer high-level resistance. Thus, PI-based regimens may be slightly more "forgiving" of less than perfect adherence—although, of course, that's probably not the message to convey to your patients.

- The PIs pose tremendous drug interaction challenges. They are all substrates of the common drug-metabolizing enzymes and thus can have their concentrations substantially increased or decreased by drugs that inhibit or induce these enzymes. Generally, coadministering other drugs that are P450 substrates (such as statins, macrolides, benzodiazepines, and calcium channel blockers) with PI regimens boosted with ritonavir or cobicistat leads to increased serum concentrations of these drugs. However, more unpredictable effects can occur, perhaps as a result of shunting to alternative pathways or mixed inhibition/induction, leading to the reduction in serum levels of P450 substrates (as can be seen with the voriconazole–ritonavir interaction). The bottom line: for patients on PIs, carefully screen all of their medications for drug interactions using the most up-to-date references.

- Ritonavir is now used almost exclusively as a pharmacokinetic booster in much lower doses than its originally approved dose of 400 mg BID. It is not well tolerated at the higher dose and the majority of prescriptions or orders for it are an error. At the least, it warrants a double-check.

What They're Good For

Darunavir-based combinations are currently among the preferred regimens for treatment of initial HIV infection, with atazanavir- or lopinavir-based combinations as an alternative. A variety of PIs are used in salvage regimens for patients with resistant virus. Their durable viral suppression needs to be balanced against their long-term toxicities (particularly cardiovascular effects), and patients should be prepared to make appropriate lifestyle changes.

Don't Forget!

Only atazanavir can be used unboosted (and this is recommended only for selected patients). If there's not a little ritonavir or cobicistat in the regimen, something is probably wrong.

Integrase Inhibitors

Agents: dolutegravir (DTG), raltegravir (RAL)

Combinations: elvitegravir/cobicistat/emtricitabine/
tenofovir disoproxil fumarate (EVG/c/FTC/TDF,
Stribild), elvitegravir/cobicistat/emtricitabine/
tenofovir alafenamide (EVG/c/FTC/TAF, Genvoya),
dolutegravir/abacavir/lamivudine (Triumeq)

The integrase inhibitors (abbreviated as INSTI for
integrase strand transfer inhibitors) went from a
"new and promising" class of antiretrovirals (*Antibiotics Simplified,* 3rd Edition!) to the anchor of
most of the preferred regimens for initial therapy.
They offer excellent tolerability, fewer drug interactions (except for elvitegravir), and one-pill, once-
daily convenience (except for raltegravir). Their
novel mechanism of action also provides a new
option for treatment-experienced patients.

Mechanism of Action

After the HIV reverse transcriptase enzyme creates a
strand of viral DNA, a viral protein called integrase
facilitates the transfer of the HIV DNA into the host
cell's genome. The INSTIs inhibit this enzyme, preventing the viral DNA from becoming a part of the
host cell enzyme, an important step in HIV replication.

Only current clinical use is for HIV.

Musculoskeletal: Raltegravir has been associated with increases in creatine phosphokinase. Most of these cases have been asymptomatic; clinically evident myositis or rhabdomyolysis is rare.

Renal: Cobicistat inhibits the renal secretion of creatinine, leading to increased levels of serum creatinine without a decline in glomerular filtration rate. It's important to differentiate this "fake" renal dysfunction from actual renal dysfunction, especially if the patient is also on tenofovir.

Important Facts

- Cobicistat isn't an antiviral, but rather a "pharmacokinetic enhancer": much like ritonavir, it is used to "boost" the concentrations of other drugs. In fact, right now elvitegravir is ONLY available in combination with cobicistat (and tenofovir and emtricitabine). Thus, concerns for drug interactions for the combination elvitegravir product are similar to those for ritonavir-boosted protease inhibitors. In contrast, raltegravir has few documented drug interactions, a considerable advantage over many antiretrovirals. Dolutegravir is more on the raltegravir end of the drug interaction spectrum, although it has enough to warrant checking your drug interaction checker on your phone (which you should do for all antiretrovirals anyway).

- A nonmetabolic drug interaction that the INS-TIs share is reduced absorption when these drugs are coadministered with divalent and tri-valent cations (the same kind of issue that flu-oroquinolones and tetracyclines display). The recommendation is that administration of the INSTI should be separated—at least 2 hours before or 6 hours after oral administration of products containing significant amounts of alu-minium, calcium, iron, magnesium, or zinc.
- The INSTIs have a relatively low genetic bar-rier to resistance, such that they would be less "forgiving" of imperfect adherence than a PI-based regimen.
- Note that elvitegravir is available as a combi-nation product with "old tenofovir" (TDF) as well as "new tenofovir" (TAF). Make sure you have the right one!

What They're Good For

As noted, these drugs have rocketed to the top of the preferred list of antiretrovirals because of their many favorable characteristics.

Don't Forget!

Because of that low genetic barrier to resistance, drug interactions that reduce INSTI levels put them at significant risk of therapeutic failure with the development of resistance. Make sure to sepa-rate from cations and run your interaction checker!

Entry and Fusion Inhibitors

While other antiretrovirals affect the HIV life cycle after infection of the cell, the entry (maraviroc) and fusion inhibitors (enfuvirtide) attempt to block HIV from infecting a cell.

Mechanism of Action

The process of HIV binding to and entering the cell involves a "handshake" between viral proteins and proteins on the host cell target. Enfuvirtide binds to a viral protein involved in fusion, while maraviroc actually targets a human protein (CCR5) that serves as a coreceptor for the virus.

Spectrum

Only current clinical use is for HIV.

Adverse Effects

Dermatologic: Injection site reactions—including pain, erythema, pruritis, and nodule formation—occur in essentially all patients using subcutaneous enfuvirtide.

Hepatotoxicity: Maraviroc has a black box warning regarding hepatotoxicity, based on case reports from healthy subjects who received the drug in early clinical trials. The effect seems to be rare in patients treated with maraviroc.

Important Facts

- Enfuvirtide is administered as a subcutaneous injection associated with substantial injection site reactions; thus, it is generally reserved for patients with the most difficult-to-treat, multidrug-resistant strains of virus.
- Because maraviroc only blocks one of two coreceptors for HIV, it will not be effective for virus strains that primarily utilize the CXCR4 coreceptor for viral entry. Hence, before a patient is started on maraviroc, a tropism test must be performed to see whether the patient's virus "prefers" CCR5 (in which case maraviroc may be useful) or CXCR4 (thus ruling out maraviroc use).
- Maraviroc is a substrate of P450 drug-metabolizing enzymes and, thus, there are different dosage recommendations depending on which other potentially interacting drugs the patient is taking.

What They're Good For

These drugs are mainly for use in treatment-experienced patients.

Don't Forget!

Before initiating maraviroc, make sure you know its "Trofile"—that is, the name of the test used to determine the pro*file* of its *trop*ism (CCR5 vs. CXCR4).

38

Antiviral Interferons

Interferons are normal human cytokines that are used by the immune system to activate cells when infection is present, fight cancerous cells, and perform other functions. They are given exogenously in the treatment of multiple diseases, ranging from multiple sclerosis to cancers to viral hepatitis. Interferon-α 2a and 2b and their pegylated forms have all been used for the treatment of both viral hepatitis B and C infections, though only pegylated forms are currently recommended.

Mechanism of Action

Interferons have multiple mechanisms of action against hepatitis B and C viruses. They have direct antiviral effects, change cellular differentiation, inhibit cell growth, activate macrophages, and increase lymphocyte cytotoxicity. Pegylated forms of interferon have had molecules of polyethylene glycol (PEG) attached to the interferon molecules to improve their pharmacokinetics by increasing their half-lives, allowing for decreased administration frequency.

Spectrum

Alpha interferons are used for the treatment of infections caused by hepatitis B virus (HBV) and hepatitis C virus (HCV).

Adverse Effects

Adverse effects are very common with interferons, leading to noncompliance, patient dropout, and avoidance of their use. Flulike symptoms are most common, including headache, fatigue, weakness, fever, and myalgia. Depression is also common and often requires pharmacologic treatment. Patients with suicidal ideation should not be given interferons. Anxiety can also occur.

Hematologic adverse effects are also common with interferons, notably cytopenias including neutropenia, anemia, and thrombocytopenia. In the treatment of HCV infection, ribavirin is usually the primary cause of anemia.

Interferons can worsen decompensated cirrhosis and are generally not administered to these patients.

Important Facts

- Pegylated interferons have supplanted non-pegylated forms for the treatment of viral hepatitis. Pegylated forms are given once weekly compared to thrice weekly for the non-pegylated interferons, improving compliance and convenience. Adverse effects are somewhat attenuated also, and efficacy is either similar or somewhat higher for the pegylated forms.
- Dosing for these agents varies significantly by agent and indication, so be cautious when prescribing or recommending them. For HCV

infection, the recommended dose of ribavirin differs for each form as well.

- For HCV infection, the two pegylated interferons have been shown to be equivalent, but their dosing is not. Pegylated interferon-α 2a is given in a fixed dose, while pegylated interferon-α 2b is dosed by weight. For HBV infection, only pegylated interferon-α 2a has an FDA indication, though pegylated interferon-α 2b has been studied as well.

- Interferons commonly cause or exacerbate depression and are contraindicated in severe depression and patients contemplating suicide. There is generally no rush in the treatment of chronic HCV infection, so ensure that your patient's depression is controlled (pharmacologically if necessary) before starting therapy. For HBV infection, other drugs are better choices in depressed patients.

What They're Good For

Since the advent of new direct-acting antiviral agents for hepatitis C, the use of interferons for this indication has declined substantially. For chronic HBV infection, nucleoside/nucleotide analogs are preferred over pegylated interferons by many clinicians (and patients) due to their much better adverse effect profile, but they are taken indefinitely compared to a finite regimen for interferon.

Don't Forget!

Watch out for the many adverse effects of interferon therapy during treatment, and be vigilant in observing for emerging depression.

Direct-Acting Anti-hepatitis C Agents

39

Agents: protease inhibitors: simeprevir, paritaprevir*, grazoprevir*, boceprevir, telaprevir*

NS5A inhibitors: daclatasvir, elbasvir*, ledipasvir*, ombitasvir*

NS5B (polymerase) inhibitors: sofosbuvir

Non-nucleoside polymerase inhibitors: dasabuvir

Combinations: paritaprevir/ombitasvir/ritonavir, grazoprevir/elbasvir, ledipasvir/sofosbuvir

The treatment of chronic hepatitis C infection has undergone as big of a revolution of therapy as HIV treatment has—but instead of unfolding over three decades, it has unfolded over 5 years.

Two serine protease inhibitors introduced in late 2011 (boceprevir, telaprevir) heralded this new era—and quickly became obsolete as more potent and better-tolerated agents have been developed. As with HIV treatment, treatment regimens using these drugs typically consist of multiple agents with different mechanisms of action. In contrast to HIV regimens, the treatment duration for these anti-HCV treatments is on the order of only 3–4 months in most patients, with cure rates ranging from 80 to 100%. Compared to prior ribavirin plus interferon-based regimens for hepatitis C, the new drugs are much better tolerated. This revolution in therapy comes at a price—as in, actual cash money price. Currently, the price of these drugs can be on the order of $1,000 *per day*. So, if you are learning about these drugs from this book—you're definitely not going to be the one who is making the decision to start therapy on a patient with them! But everyone involved in the care of these patients has important roles to play in ensuring compliance, screening for drug interactions, and monitoring for potential adverse effects.

Mechanism of Action

Along with ribavirin, these agents are considered to be direct-acting antivirals (DAAs)—to distinguish them from the indirect anti-HCV effects of interferon. Their mechanisms are varied; some inhibit proteases, others RNA polymerases (NS5B protein—"NS" stands for "non-structural"), and in the case of the NS5A inhibitors—it's not exactly clear how they work. Following the model of the latest HIV therapies, most of the agents are co-formulated in fixed combinations, which reduces the need to select drugs with different mechanisms "from the menu."

Spectrum

There are at least 6 HCV genotypes that can cause infection in humans and the DAAs differ in their activity against each. Genotype 1 (which comes in 1a and 1b flavors) is the most prevalent in the United States and as such each of the current regimens has activity against these. Protease inhibitors have potent activity against genotype-1 agents, but simeprevir and paritaprevir have limited activity against other genotypes. NS5A and NS5B inhibitors have a broad spectrum of activity against various HCV genotypes. Note that ritonavir is co-formulated with ombitasvir and paritaprevir solely as a pharmacokinetic booster, not because of any anti-HCV activity.

Adverse Effects

Besides their potent activity, the substantially greater tolerability of these drugs relative to ribavirin and interferon is responsible for their having rapidly become the regimens of choice. Most agents are well tolerated and typically associated with mild toxicities, including nausea, vomiting, and fatigue.

Simeprevir is associated with photosensitivity and thus patients should limit sun exposure and/or wear sunscreen while taking this medication. Transient elevations in bilirubin are frequently seen but do not appear to be associated with significant hepatotoxicity.

Sofosbuvir is rarely associated with symptomatic episodes of bradycardia, but almost all of these occurred in the context of patients receiving concomitant amiodarone.

Elbasvir/grazoprevir and ombitasvir/paritaprevir/ritonavir have been associated with hepatic decompensation in some patients, particularly those with pre-existing cirrhosis. Close monitoring of ALT is indicated, with treatment interruption recommended for substantial asymptomatic elevations (e.g., >10-fold of upper limit of normal) or lower elevations that are associated with symptoms of hepatitis (e.g., jaundice, nausea, vomiting, abdominal pain).

Important Facts

- These agents have LOTS of drug interactions, and given the high prevalence of HIV–HCV coinfection, interactions with antiretrovirals are a major issue. The interactions are mediated through cytochrome P450 metabolism, as well as by interference with transporters like P-glycoprotein or the organic anion transporters. The Website http://www.hep-druginteractions .org is an excellent resource for assessing drug interactions of DAAs with a wide spectrum of agents, including antiretrovirals.
- Administration with food can be an important consideration for some of these agents: simeprevir, ombitasivir/paritaprevir/ritonavir, and dasabuvir are recommended to be administered with food. Also, the presence of gastric acidity is important for the absorption of ledipasvir; thus, patients who receive the ledipasvir/sofosbuvir combination should avoid acid-suppressing agents or carefully time their administration with respect to ledipasvir/sofosbuvir.
- For some genotypes and patient populations (e.g., cirrhotic patients), addition of ribavirin or pegylated interferon to the DAA regimen is still recommended.
- Resistance to these agents does emerge during therapy and seems to correlate with failure to

eradicate HCV. The genetic barrier for resistance emergence is lowest with dasabuvir, the NS5A inhibitors, and simeprevir and higher with the other protease inhibitors and sofosbuvir. The clinical significance of resistance mutations to DAAs is less well established than for HIV antiretrovirals. Thus, testing for the presence of resistance mutations is recommended before initiating therapy only in selected patients, including those with prior exposure to DAAs and some patients with cirrhosis.

What They're Good For

These drugs are used in the treatment of patients with chronic HCV infection, where they are typically associated with a high rate of cure.

Don't Forget!

These drugs represent a true breakthrough in treating HCV, but the drugs are expensive (meaning they may only get one shot at therapy) and drug interactions are problematic, so patients need all the help they can get to make sure they get the most out of their treatment course.

40

Ribavirin

Agent: ribavirin

Ribavirin is an antiviral agent that is active against many different types of viruses, though it is used primarily for the treatment of HCV and respiratory syncytial virus (RSV) infection. The addition of ribavirin to some other agents for HCV treatment increases both the effectiveness and toxicity of treatment.

Mechanism of Action

The mechanism of action of ribavirin is not well characterized, but it is a nucleoside analogue of guanosine that is phosphorylated into its active form inside cells. Technically it is a direct-acting anti-HCV antiviral like those discussed in Chapter 39, but is generally considered separately from those agents.

Spectrum

Well-characterized activity has been described for HCV and RSV, though ribavirin has some activity against other viruses as well including influenza and adenovirus.

Adverse Effects

The main adverse effect of ribavirin is haemolytic anemia. This effect is dose-related, dose-limiting, and may be severe. Interferons, which are often administered with oral ribavirin for treatment of HCV, can exacerbate this effect because they cause cytopenias as well. Ribavirin is also associated with fatigue, headaches, and insomnia, though it is difficult to determine whether ribavirin itself, interferons, or the combination are responsible. In practice it does not matter as the effects must be managed during combination therapy.

Important Facts

- For the treatment of HCV infection, ribavirin must always be used in combination. As mono-therapy, ribavirin rapidly leads to resistant-mutants of HCV.
- Ribavirin is usually administered orally, but it can also be given in an aerosolized form to patients with pulmonary RSV infection, princi-pally in young children and in immunocompro-mised adults, most notably patients with lung or hematopoietic stem cell transplants. Admin-istration via this route is technically complex, since efforts need to be made to reduce the environmental exposure of ribavirin—a known teratogen. Recent studies suggest that orally administered ribavirin may be similarly effec-tive, and many centers are moving away from inhaled administration, at least in adults.
- Ribavirin causes birth defects and is pregnancy category X. Fertile women taking ribavirin should use reliable contraception. Pregnant

women must also avoid aerosolized ribavirin and pregnant healthcare workers should avoid caring for patients receiving it, if possible.

- The primary means of managing ribavirin-induced anemia is dose reduction. If anemia becomes severe or persistent, erythropoietin can be given.

What It's Good For

Ribavirin is used as part of combination therapies for some patients with HCV chronic infection. Ribavirin (aerosolized or oral) is used to treat severe RSV in both children and adults, primarily immunocompromised patients or those with severe comorbidities.

Don't Forget!

Hemoglobin concentrations must be closely watched during ribavirin therapy. Expect some degree of anemia to occur and be prepared to act accordingly.

41

Hepatitis B Nucleoside Analogs

Agents: entecavir, adefovir, telbivudine

Analogs of viral nucleosides are useful not just for the treatment of HIV infection, but for HBV infection as well. Because HBV is a DNA virus, these drugs can compete for viral enzymes with native viral nucleosides just as they do for reverse transcriptase in HIV. Several of them are active in both HIV and HBV infection, an obvious bonus for patients who are infected with both viruses. All are easy-to-take drugs that have changed the management of HBV to offer an interferon-free regimen that is prolonged, but well tolerated. Several HIV nucleoside/tide reverse transcriptase inhibitors are also used to treat HBV, and tenofovir is a drug of choice in both disease states.

Mechanism of Action

Nucleoside analogs inhibit the action of viral DNA polymerase by taking the place of nucleotides in the elongating strand of viral DNA, leading to early termination of the viral DNA strain.

Spectrum

These drugs are active against HBV and HIV, though they are not primarily used for HIV infection.

Adverse Effects

These agents are all very well tolerated by most patients and have a low incidence of adverse effects. Fatigue and elevations in creatinine phosphokinase are possible, though the latter may be associated with HBV itself. Lactic acidosis is uncommon.

Important Facts

- All of these drugs have some activity against HIV, though the doses that are required to treat HIV infection are higher than the HBV doses. Using them at the lower HBV doses in an HIV/HBV coinfected patient can select for mutant viruses that are resistant to NRTIs and this should be avoided. Patients with known HBV should be tested for HIV before therapy is started with one of these drugs.
- Whenever a drug that is active in both HIV and HBV is used, like lamivudine or tenofovir (both NRTIs), it should be given in the higher HIV dose.

What They're Good For

Along with tenofovir, these are drugs of choice for chronic HBV infection. They do not cure the infection, but can repress it to the point that it does not progress.

Don't Forget!

Be sure your patient is not coinfected with HIV before treating HBV with one of these drugs.

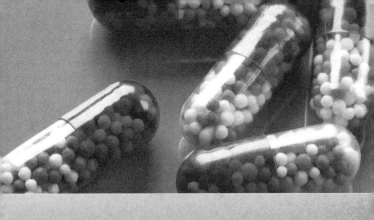

Antiparasitic Drugs

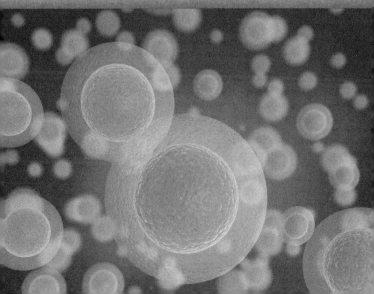

PART 6

Antiparasitic Drugs

Introduction to Antiparasitic Drugs

There is a tremendously unequal variation in the human burden of parasitic disease, based on geography, industrialization/hygiene, and immune status. It is estimated that up to half of the world's population is chronically infected with parasites. The extent of parasite-related morbidity and mortality depends on parasite burden, preexisting immunity, and patient comorbidities. We focus on parasitic diseases primarily affecting inhabitants of industrialized nations. Parasites causing human disease can be broadly grouped into two main categories, the unicellular protozoa and the multicellular helminthes (Table 42–1). The protozoa have many subgroups, but we present them as primarily intestinal or primarily extraintestinal pathogens. The helminthes are subdivided into nematodes (roundworms), trematodes (flukes), and cestodes (tapeworms). Examples of common pathogens for each group are given along with some of the agents used in their treatment. Although not technically considered parasites, two other organisms that are susceptible to antiparasitic drugs also are addressed: *Pneumocystis jirovecii* (technically a fungus) and *Sarcoptes scabiei* (the scabies mite, technically an Arachnid).

TABLE 42–1

Grouping of Parasites with Commonly Encountered Pathogens and Commonly Used Antiparasitic Agents

Group	Subgroup	Examples	Antiparasitics*
Protozoa	Extraintestinal	*Plasmodium* (malaria)	**Quinolines** Doxycycline
		Toxoplasma	Clindamycin **Atovaquone-proguanil** *Arteminsins* Pyrimethamine/ Sulfadiazine TMP/SMX
		Trypansoma	**Pentamidine**
	Intestinal	*Entamoeba* *Giardia* *Cryptosporidium*	Metronidazole Tinidazole Paromomycin
Helminths	Nematodes	*Ascaris* *Strongyloides*	**Albendazole** **Ivermectin** *Praziquantel* **Albendazole** *Praziquantel*
	Trematodes	*Schistosoma*	
	Cestodes	*Echinococcus* *Taenia*	
Other organisms	Fungus	*Pneumocystis*	TMP/SMX Clindamycin/ **Primaquine** **Atovaquone** **Pentamidine**
	Ectoparasites	Scabies	**Ivermectin**

*Agents in **bold** are discussed in this section; agents in normal type are covered in other chapters; agents in *italics* are not discussed in this book.

Drugs with antiparasitic activity range from everyday antibacterial drugs (metronidazole, doxycycline) to mildly exciting agents seen occasionally in routine practice (chloroquine, pentamidine) to the most exotic agents that can be obtained only from the Centers for Disease Control and Prevention (CDC) in the United States (diethylcarbamazine, sodium stibogluconate). In this part we will focus on the middle category, leaving the details of antibacterial drugs to their own chapters and the exotic agents to those with a keen interest.

Quinolines

43

Agents: chloroquine, mefloquine, quinidine, quinine, primaquine, amodiaquine, hydroxychloroquine

The quinoline agents are among the oldest anti-infective agents used by humans, with recorded use of the bark of the *Cinchona* tree (imported from Peru) to treat fever in malarious areas of Europe dating back to the seventeenth century. The primary component of this remedy was quinine, the first antimalarial agent to be widely used. Although malaria is no longer endemic to most industrialized countries, it is considered to be the most important cause of fever in returning travelers, especially those not native to endemic areas, because of the potential for severe illness. There are important differences between the quinolines in activity based on both the species of *Plasmodium* and the geographic area; readers are advised to consult their updated national guidelines when managing suspected malaria cases.

Mechanism of Action

The mechanisms of action of quinolines on parasites are incompletely understood. Chloroquine, quinine, and quinidine appear to interfere with the ability of the malaria parasite to detoxify hemo-globin metabolites. Primaquine appears to affect parasitic mitochondrial function.

Spectrum

Protozoa (activity variable by region): Plasmodium falciparum, Plasmodium malariae, Plasmodium ovale, Plasmodium vivax

Like-a-parasite-but-technically-a-fungus: Pneumocystis jirovecii (primaquine)

Adverse Effects

Cardiovascular: The quinolines can cause dose-related cardiovascular toxicity, including QT interval prolongation, hypotension, and potentially fatal ventricular arrhythmias. Quinidine is a class IA antiarrhythmic, and it is also used therapeutically in the treatment of some arrhythmias (however, like many antiarrhythmics, it can be proarrhythmic). Cardiovascular effects are most likely with IV quinidine; less common with quinine, mefloquine, and chloroquine; and rare with primaquine.

Hematologic: Primaquine can cause hemolysis in patients deficient in glucose-6-phosphate dehydrogenase (G6PD); testing for G6PD deficiency is required before use.

Metabolic: Quinidine and quinine can cause profound hypoglycemia resulting from the stimulated release of insulin.

Psychiatric: Mefloquine is associated with a range of psychiatric disturbances ranging from insomnia, vivid dreams, and mood swings to depression, psychosis, and suicide. Although mefloquine is well tolerated by the vast majority of patients taking the drug, patients with a history of psychiatric issues, including depression, should avoid taking mefloquine.

Systemic: The syndrome of "cinchonism" (tinnitus, headache, nausea, and visual disturbances) is common in patients receiving therapeutic doses of quinine. These effects can lead to discontinuation of therapy because of intolerance, but they resolve after drug discontinuation.

Important Facts

- In the United States, quinidine is the only quinoline available intravenously. It is used in combination regimens for treatment of severe malaria. Intensive monitoring, including continuous monitoring of blood pressure and electrocardiogram (ECG) and serial monitoring of blood glucose, is required. The dosing of quinidine is altered in renal failure, which is not uncommon in severe malaria.
- Unlike other antimalarial drugs, primaquine is active against the "hypnozoite" forms of *P. vivax* and *P. ovale* that can lay dormant in the liver and cause relapsing infections. Thus, a 2-week course of primaquine is added to the antimalarial regimen when infection with these species is documented.

What They're Good For

Chloroquine: Treatment of uncomplicated malaria acquired in chloroquine-sensitive areas (only a few regions) and prophylaxis against malaria in travelers to those regions

Mefloquine: Treatment of uncomplicated malaria acquired in mefloquine-sensitive areas (most of the world except Southeast Asia) and prophylaxis against malaria in travelers to those regions

Quinine/quinidine: Treatment of severe malaria (quinidine) in combination with doxycycline, tetracycline, or clindamycin; not used for prophylaxis

Primaquine: Treatment of uncomplicated malaria due to *P. vivax* or *P. ovale* in combination with a second agent, prophylaxis against malaria in travelers where *P. vivax* is the principal species, in combination with clindamycin, and in treatment of mild-to-moderate *Pneumocystis* pneumonia

Don't Forget!

As with bacterial infections, the progression of antimicrobial resistance makes treatment of and prophylaxis against malaria difficult. Because most clinicians deal with malaria infrequently, there is no shame in double-checking national guidelines to make sure you are using the most appropriate regimen for your patient. The CDC even has a malaria hotline to help clinicians deal with treatment of cases [business hours (855) 856-4713; after hours (770) 488-7788].

44

Atovaquone

Atovaquone is an antiparasitic agent with activity against several important protozoans. Its activity against the malaria parasite is enhanced when given in combination with the drug proguanil (this co-formulated tablet is known as Malarone). Atovaquone tends to be better tolerated than comparator drugs but is limited by the lack of an IV formulation (for severe disease), high cost, and somewhat lower efficacy (for *Pneumocystis* disease).

Mechanism of Action

Atovaquone appears to interfere with electron transport in the parasitic mitochondria.

Spectrum

Like-a-parasite-but-technically-a-fungus: Pneumocystis jirovecii

Protozoa: Plasmodium species, *Toxoplasma gondii*, *Babesia* species

Adverse Effects

Both atovaquone and atovaquone/proguanil are very well tolerated. The most common adverse effects are gastrointestinal (nausea/vomiting, diarrhea, abdominal pain).

▨ Important Facts

- Atovaquone is available as a suspension, while atovaquone/proguanil is formulated as a tablet. Bioavailability is rather low with both, but it is enhanced substantially when given with food, especially high-fat meals. Both agents should be administered with food.

- In clinical trials of atovaquone in treating mild-to-moderate *Pneumocystis* pneumonia in patients intolerant of TMP/SMX, atovaquone was slightly less effective than its comparators (dapsone or pentamidine) but better tolerated, leading to similar overall success rates. Atovaquone should not be used in patients with severe *Pneumocystis* pneumonia or in patients whose GI absorption is thought to be poor.

- Other than its cost, atovaquone/proguanil is a favorable drug for malaria prophylaxis for travelers. It is highly effective, well tolerated, active against chloroquine-resistant *Plasmodium*, and requires administration only 1–2 days prior to travel, while in the malaria-endemic area, and for 7 days after return. Many other agents used for malaria prophylaxis require beginning the medication 2 weeks before travel and continuing for 4 weeks afterward.

What They're Good For

Atovaquone: Treatment of mild-to-moderate *Pneumocystis* pneumonia and prophylaxis against *Pneumocystis* in patients intolerant of first-line therapy

Atovaquone/proguanil: Treatment of uncomplicated malaria and prophylaxis against malaria

Don't Forget!

Make sure your patients take their atovaquone with food (or at the very least a glass of milk); the bioavailability of atovaquone is increased approximately five times when administered with food compared with the fasting state.

45

Benzimidazoles

Agents: albendazole, mebendazole, thiabendazole

These drugs are used primarily to treat infections caused by helminthes (worms), ranging from the common pinworms found in children to pathogens causing massive cystic lesions in the brain. Most intestinal worm infections can be cured with a single dose of these drugs; for tissue-invasive disease, prolonged courses are necessary. Note that mebendazole and thiabendazole are no longer available in the United States.

Mechanism of Action

The benzimidazoles interfere with elongation of the microtubules that are responsible for parasitic cellular structure, leading to a disruption of growth and division.

Spectrum

Nematodes (roundworms): Ascaris lumbricoides (roundworm), *Enterobius vermicularis* (pinworm), *Necator americanus* (hookworm), *Strongyloides stercoralis* (threadworm)

Cestodes (tapeworms): Echinococcus (liver abscess), *Taenia solium* (neurocysticercosis)

Adverse Effects

Albendazole is very well tolerated, especially when used as single-dose therapy in treatment of intestinal worm infection. With multidose regimens, adverse effects are primarily gastrointestinal, although hepatotoxicity and neutropenia are rarely reported. Thiabendazole is the most toxic and can cause CNS adverse effects. These drugs should generally be avoided in pregnancy, although some data suggest that they may be safe after the first trimester.

Important Facts

- Although data are limited, these drugs appear to be substrates of the cytochrome P450 system. Thus, it is possible that coadministration with strong inducers of drug-metabolizing enzymes such as phenytoin and rifampin may lower serum levels. Oral absorption of albendazole is limited, which generally does not pose a problem for treatment of intestinal nematode infections, and thus drug interactions would not be of concern. However, in treatment of systemic infections, caution is advised with coadministration of enzyme-inducing agents because of the potential for subtherapeutic drug levels.

What They're Good For

As a single-dose therapy of most intestinal nematode infections, as an alternative for treatment of *Strongyloides* infection, and as treatment for tissue-invasive *Echinococcus* or *Taenia* infection.

Don't Forget!

For some parasitic infections, drug-induced killing of the parasite releases antigens that can cause allergic reactions. Corticosteroids are sometimes administered to mitigate this effect. Know which infections this applies to before using antiparasitics for invasive infections.

46

Pentamidine

Agent: pentamidine

Pentamidine is the primary alternative to trimethoprim/sulfamethoxazole (TMP/SMX) for patients with *Pneumocystis* pneumonia, which was once an extremely common cause of severe pneumonia in HIV-infected patients but is becoming less common with effective antiretroviral therapy. It is also very toxic, so familiarity with its extensive adverse effects is required. It can be given either intravenously or by inhalation, and the proper route depends upon the indication.

Mechanism of Action

Pentamidine appears to bind to and disrupt the function of transfer RNA, resulting in inhibition of protein synthesis.

Spectrum

Like-a-parasite-but-technically-a-fungus: Pneumocystis jirovecii
Protozoa: Trypanosoma, Leishmania

Adverse Effects (IV pentamidine)

Cardiovascular: Hypotension can occur with rapid infusion of pentamidine; the drug should be infused over at least an hour. Cases of QT prolongation with ventricular arrhythmia have also been reported.

Metabolic: Pentamidine is toxic to the pancreas, leading to dysglycemias in up to 25% of patients. The course of this toxicity may initially manifest as hypoglycemia because pentamidine-induced pancreatic injury causes release of insulin from islet cells. Later, continuing injury can cause a decrease in pancreatic function, with hypo-insulinemia and hyperglycemia. Continued use may lead to irreversible damage, leaving patients with diabetes mellitus. Other manifestations of pancreatitis may also occur.

Renal: Nephrotoxicity is common with pentamidine, although it is generally reversible upon drug discontinuation. Electrolyte disturbances, including hypokalemia and hypocalcemia, may also occur.

Respiratory: Administration of pentamidine as an inhalation may induce bronchoconstriction, especially in patients with asthma. Pretreatment with an inhaled bronchodilator may attenuate these effects.

Important Facts

- In clinical trials of pentamidine as treatment for *Pneumocystis* pneumonia, pentamidine appeared to be about equal in efficacy to TMP/SMX; however, only about half of patients could tolerate a full course of IV pentamidine without discontinuing the drug or decreasing the dose. Careful monitoring (ECG, metabolic panel) and supportive care interventions (electrolyte replacement, glucose, or insulin as appropriate) are necessary. Also, dosage adjustment in patients with renal insufficiency is recommended.

- Once-monthly inhaled pentamidine has reasonable efficacy as a second-line agent for prophylaxis against *Pneumocystis* pneumonia. However, unlike with TMP/SMX prophylaxis, cases of extrapulmonary *Pneumocystis* infection have been reported in patients on inhaled pentamidine. Inhaled pentamidine also does not protect against *Toxoplasma* disease or bacterial pneumonia as TMP/SMX does.

What It's Good For

IV pentamidine is an alternative drug for treatment of severe *Pneumocystis* pneumonia; inhaled pentamidine is an alternative for prophylaxis against *Pneumocystis* pneumonia. IV pentamidine is an alternative drug for treatment of leishmaniasis and trypanosomiasis.

Don't Forget!

Watch out for overlapping toxicities with pentamidine and other drugs the patient may be on. Patients receiving pentamidine are often severely ill and may be on drugs like insulin, furosemide, aminoglycosides, and antiarrhythmics that may exacerbate pentamidine's myriad adverse effects.

47

Ivermectin

If you practice in a healthcare institution, you will likely be treated to at least one scabies outbreak over your career, if not one each year. While scabies is most often treated with permethrin cream, patients or their healthcare providers who are unable or unwilling to baste themselves in the cream will receive oral ivermectin. Ivermectin is also given to patients with the highly contagious "Norwegian scabies" (an unwarranted aspersion on Scandinavian hygiene). In addition to scabies, ivermectin is also effective in treating several diseases that may be endemic in tropical settings, such as the causative agents of river blindness, strongyloidiasis, and cutaneous larva migrans, the latter two of which occur, if infrequently, in the United States. It can also be used for treatment of *Strongyloides* hyperinfection syndrome, an increasingly recognized cause of life-threatening illness in immunocompromised patients.

Mechanism of Action

Ivermectin binds to the parasitic neuromuscular junction, causing muscular paralysis of the parasite. The parasite dies directly from the effects or from starvation.

Spectrum

Ectoparasites: Sarcoptes scabiei (scabies mite),
Pediculus humanus (lice)

Nematodes (roundworms): Onchocerca volvulus
(river blindness), *Strongyloides stercoralis*
(strongyloidiasis), *Ancylostoma braziliense*
(cutaneous larva migrans), other nematodes

Adverse Effects

In treatment of scabies, ivermectin is very well tolerated. Severe adverse reactions, including fever, myalgia, and hypotension, have been reported when ivermectin is used for management of nematode infections in endemic settings. These effects are thought to be a result of the host's immune response to antigens released from killed parasites. These effects are more severe in patients with higher worm burdens, and they generally resolve soon after drug administration.

Important Facts

- Yes, ivermectin is the same drug you use to treat your dog's heartworms. It is also at the center of a heart*worming* story: after ivermectin was shown to be effective as a once-yearly treatment for river blindness, the pharmaceutical company Merck offered to donate—free of charge—as much ivermectin as was needed to treat the disease. It is estimated that 200-million free treatments have been provided to date, avoiding more than half a million cases of blindness. Hey, at this point in the book, we figured you could use some good news (and bad puns).

What It's Good For

Ivermectin is used as an alternative to topical permethrin for scabies infection, to topical therapies for treatment of head or body louse infestation, and for treatment of *Ancylostoma* infections. It is also a drug of choice for infection caused by *Strongyloides* or *Onchocerca*.

Don't Forget!

For treatment of ectoparasitic (scabies or lice) infestation, ivermectin should be administered as two doses, approximately 1 week apart. Administration of a single dose increases the risk of relapse.

Selected Normal Human Flora

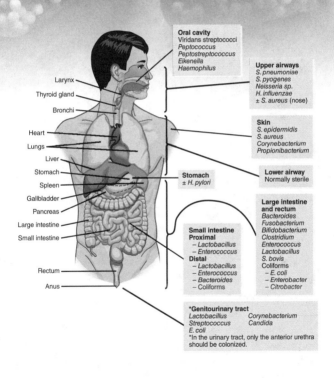

Oral cavity
Viridans streptococci
Peptococcus
Peptostreptococcus
Eikenella
Haemophilus

Upper airways
S. pneumoniae
S. pyogenes
Neisseria sp.
H. influenzae
± *S. aureus* (nose)

Skin
S. epidermidis
S. aureus
Corynebacterium
Propionibacterium

Lower airway
Normally sterile

Stomach
± *H. pylori*

**Large intestine
and rectum**
Bacteroides
Fusobacterium
Bifidobacterium
Clostridium
Enterococcus
Lactobacillus
S. bovis
Coliforms
– *E. coli*
– *Enterobacter*
– *Citrobacter*

Small intestine
Proximal
 – *Lactobacillus*
 – *Enterococcus*
Distal
 – *Lactobacillus*
 – *Enterococcus*
 – *Bacteroides*
 – Coliforms

Larynx
Thyroid gland
Bronchi
Heart
Lungs
Liver
Stomach
Spleen
Gallbladder
Pancreas
Large intestine
Small intestine
Rectum
Anus

*Genitourinary tract
Lactobacillus   *Corynebacterium*
Streptococcus   *Candida*
E. coli
*In the urinary tract, only the anterior urethra
should be colonized.

Spectrum of Activity

Spectrum of activity is usually thought of as "does this drug cover this bug?" It is important to realize that this is a substantial oversimplification. A more accurate statement would be, "What is the probability, in this patient, that the pathogen I am concerned about is susceptible *in vitro* to this antibiotic?" The key components are "probability" and "in this patient." Some antibiotics are *always* active against some organisms (e.g., penicillin and *Streptococcus pyogenes*) and a fair number of antibiotics are *never* active against some organisms at safe concentrations (e.g., vancomycin and *Escherichia coli*). But it is more common that there is some degree of variability in susceptibility across different isolates of the organism, and that there is variability in this variability! For example, Table A–1 describes the susceptibility of *E. coli* to ciprofloxacin at three hospitals—Major Medical Center, Trauma Hospital, and the Regional Children's Hospital—all located in the same city (this example is based on actual data, but the names have been changed to protect the "innocent" institutions).

TABLE A–1

Susceptibility of *E. coli* to Ciprofloxacin at Three Hospitals

Antimicrobial	Organism	Year	Site	% Susceptible
Ciprofloxacin	*E. coli*	1998	Major Medical Center: Adults	96.3
Ciprofloxacin	*E. coli*	2008	Major Medical Center: Adults	58.0
Ciprofloxacin	*E. coli*	2008	Trauma Hospital	85.0
Ciprofloxacin	*E. coli*	2008	Regional Children's Hospital	94.0

One key aspect of variability is time: you can see that in 1998, ciprofloxacin had excellent activity against *E. coli* isolated from inpatients at Major Medical Center. Over the next decade, its activity declined sharply. So it is important to keep "when" in perspective when reading the literature about spectrum of activity; sadly, the general trend is for susceptibility to decrease over time. Another aspect of variability is "where." Trauma Hospital is just on the other side of town from Major Medical Center, but among patients there, ciprofloxacin is much more active. There can be substantial geographic variability in susceptibility in different countries, states, regions, and even, as illustrated here, within a city. Although the variability in this case is most related to the last consideration, "who," as illustrated by the excellent activity of ciprofloxacin against *E. coli* among patients at the Regional Children's Hospital. Regional Children's Hospital is located *within* the Major Medical Center, so it is not a matter of geography *per se*. Those patients are less likely to be exposed to fluoroquinolones and thus less likely to develop and spread resistant organisms to each other. So to best answer the question, "Does ciprofloxacin cover *E. coli* in this city?", you want to know when the data were collected, where the patient acquired the infection, and who the patient is (in terms of risk factors for resistance).

With that caution, no one can hold all of the different percentage susceptibilities for different drug–bug combinations in their heads, so learning general patterns of susceptibility is the first step. Tables A–2 and A–3 represent the *usual* (average across most areas and patient populations), *clinically useful* (not just good in the test tube) spectrum of activity for antibiotics and antifungal for *empiric* use.

TABLE A-2
Clinically Useful Spectra of Activity for Empiric Antibiotic Selection

	MSSA	MRSA	Strep	Enterococci	GNR	Pseudo	Anaerobes*	Atypicals
Penicillin G			++	+				
Ampicillin			++	++	+			
Amp/Sulb	++		++	++	+		++	
Pip/Tazo	++		++	++	++	++	++	
Cefazolin	++		++		+			
Cefuroxime	+		+		++			
Cefotetan	+		+		++		+	
Ceftriaxone	+		++		++			
Ceftazidime					++	++		
Cefepime	+		++		++	++		
Ceftaroline	++	++	++		++			
Aztreonam					++	++		
Imi/Mero/Dori	++		++	+	++	++	++	

Ertapenem	++				++		‡	
Gent/Tobra	(syn†)	+/-		(syn†)	(syn†)	++		
Ciprofloxacin	+/-		++		++	+		‡
Levofloxacin	++		++	+/-	++	+		‡
Moxifloxacin	++		+	+/-	++		+	‡
Doxycycline	+	+/-	+	+/-	+			‡
Tigecycline	++	++	++	++	++		‡	‡
Clindamycin	++	+	++				+	
Vancomycin	++	++	++	++				
Azithromycin	+/-		+				‡	‡
Metronidazole								‡
Telithromycin	+		++		+			‡
Daptomycin	++	++	++	++				
Linezolid	++	++	++	++				
Quin/Dalf	++	++	++	++				

(Continues)

TABLE A-2
Clinically Useful Spectra of Activity for Empiric Antibiotic Selection (*Continued*)

	MSSA	MRSA	Strep	Enterococci	GNR	Pseudo	Anaerobes*	Atypicals
Nitrofurantoin				+	+			
Fosfomycin				+	++	+		
TMP/SMX	++	+	+/−		+			

Key: ++ = good activity; + = some activity; +/− = variable activity

*Anerobes here include GI anerobes except *Clostridium difficile*, for which the only antibiotics with good clinical activity on this list are vancomycin and metronidazole.

†Aminoglycosides have useful synergistic activity versus Gram-positive cocci only when paired with a cell-wall active agent (e.g., beta-lactams, vancomycin).

Abbreviations: MSSA = methicillin-sensitive *Staphylococcus aureus*; MRSA = methicillin-resistant *Staphylococcus aureus*; Strep = streptococci; GNR = aerobic Gram-negative rods (in general, and not including *Pseudomonas aeruginosa*); Pseudo = *Pseudomonas aeruginosa*; Imi/Mero/Dori=imipenem, meropenem, doripenem; Gent/Tobra=gentamicin, tobramycin; Amp/Sulb = ampicillin/sulbactam; Pip/Tazo = piperacillin/tazobactam; Quin/Dalf = quinupristin/dalfopristin; TMP/SMX = trimethoprim/sulfamethoxazole.

TABLE A-3
Clinically Useful Spectra of Activity for Empiric Antifungal Selection

	Candida albicans, C. parapsilosis, C. tropicalis	Candida glabrata	Candida krusei	Cryptococcus	Aspergillus	Mucorales
Fluconazole	++	+/−		++		
Itraconazole	++	+/−	+/−	++	+	
Voriconazole	++	+	+	++	++	
Posaconazole/ isavuconazole	++	+	+	++	++	+
Amphotericin	++	+	++	++	++	‡
Anidula/Caspo/ Mica	++	++	++		+	

Key: ++ = good activity; + = some activity; +/− = variable activity
Abbreviation: Anidula/Caspo/Mica = anidulafungin, caspofungin, micafungin.

Infection	Common Pathogens	Patient/Infection Factors	Initial Empiric Therapy Options
Community-acquired pneumonia	Streptococcus pneumoniae Haemophilus influenzae Mycoplasma pneumoniae Chlamydophila pneumoniae Legionella pneumophila	Outpatient, otherwise healthy, no recent antibiotic exposure	Doxycycline or Azithromycin or Clarithromycin
		Outpatient, comorbidities and/or recent antibiotic exposure	Amoxicillin or Amoxicillin/Clavulanate or Cefuroxime -Plus- Azithromycin or Clarithromycin -OR- Levofloxacin or Moxifloxacin or Gemifloxacin

(Continues)

Infection	Common Pathogens	Patient/Infection Factors	Initial Empiric Therapy Options
		Inpatient, non-ICU	Ceftriaxone or Cefotaxime or Ampicillin or Ertapenem -Plus- Azithromycin or Clarithromycin or Doxycycline -OR- Levofloxacin or Moxifloxacin
		Inpatient, ICU	Ceftriaxone or Cefotaxime or Ampicillin/Sulbactam -Plus- Azithromycin or Levofloxacin or Moxifloxacin
Healthcare-associated pneumonia	*Streptococcus pneumoniae* *Haemophilus influenzae* *Staphylococcus aureus* (MSSA) *Escherichia coli* *Klebsiella pnueumoniae*	Early-onset (within 5 days of hospitalization) and no recent antibiotic exposure	Ceftriaxone or Ampicillin/Sulbactam or Ertapenem or Levofloxacin or Moxifloxacin

	Late-onset (after 5 days of hospitalization) and/or recent antibiotic exposure	Cefepime or Ceftazidime or Imipenem or Meropenem or Piperacillin/Tazobactam or Aztreonam
		-*Plus*-
		Ciprofloxacin or Levofloxacin or Gentamicin or Tobramycin or Amikacin
		-*Plus*-
		Vancomycin or Linezolid
Otitis media	Mild-moderate otalgia with temperature ≤ 39°C	Amoxicillin or Cefuroxime or Cefpodoxime or Azithromycin
	Severe otalgia and/or temperature ≥ 39°C	Amoxicillin/Clavulanate or Ceftriaxone

As above plus:
Staphylococcus aureus (MRSA)
Enterobacter species
Proteus species
Serratia species
Pseudomonas aeruginosa

Viruses
Streptococcus pneumoniae
Haemophilus influenzae
Moraxella catarrhalis

(*Continues*)

Infection	Common Pathogens	Patient/Infection Factors	Initial Empiric Therapy Options
Pharyngitis	Viruses *Streptococcus pyogenes*	Documented or high risk for *Streptococcus pyogenes*	Penicillin VK or Cephalexin or Azithromycin
Urinary tract infections	*Escherichia coli* *Proteus* species *Klebsiella pneumoniae* *Staphylococcus saprophyticus* *Enterococcus* species	Uncomplicated community-acquired lower urinary tract infection in healthy women, < 50 years old	TMP/SMX or Nitrofurantoin or Fosfomycin or Ciprofloxacin or Levofloxacin
		Community-acquired complicated urinary tract infection or pyelonephritis	Ciprofloxacin or Levofloxacin or Ceftriaxone or Ertapenem
	As above plus: *Enterobacter* species *Pseudomonas aeruginosa*	Nosocomial complicated urinary tract infection or pyelonephritis	Ceftazidime or Piperacillin/Tazobactam or Cefepime or Meropenem or Imipenem
Skin/soft tissue infections	*Streptococcus pyogenes* *Staphylococcus aureus*	Low risk for MRSA	Cefazolin or Nafcillin or Cephalexin or Dicloxacillin
		High risk for MRSA	Vancomycin or Linezolid or Clindamycin *–OR–* Cephalexin or Dicloxacillin *–Plus–* Doxycycline or TMP/SMX

	As above plus: *Escherichia coli* *Proteus* species *Klebsiella pneumoniae* *Bacteroides fragilis* *Enterococcus* species *Pseudomonas aeruginosa*	Diabetic foot infection, moderate to severe	Ceftriaxone or Ampicillin/Sulbactam or Piperacillin/Tazobactam or Ertapenem -OR- Levofloxacin or Ciprofloxacin -Plus- Clindamycin All WITH or WITHOUT Vancomycin
Intra-abdominal infections	*Escherichia coli* *Proteus* species *Klebsiella pneumoniae* *Bacteroides fragilis* *Enterococcus* species viridans *Streptococcus*	Community-acquired, mild-moderate severity	Ertapenem or Moxifloxacin or Tigecycline -OR- Cefazolin or Ceftriaxone or Levofloxacin or Ciprofloxacin -Plus- Metronidazole
	As above plus: *Pseudomonas aeruginosa* *Enterobacter spp* *Serratia spp*	Community-acquired, high severity or high-risk patient -OR- Nosocomial (any severity or patient)	Piperacillin/Tazobactam or Imipenem or Meropenem -OR- Ceftazidime or Cefepime -Plus- Metronidazole All WITH or WITHOUT Vancomycin

(Continues)

Infection	Common Pathogens	Patient/Infection Factors	Initial Empiric Therapy Options
Community-acquired meningitis	*Streptococcus pneumoniae* *Neisseria meningitidis*	Otherwise healthy, 2–50 years of age	Ceftriaxone -Plus- Vancomycin
	As above plus: *Listeria monocytogenes*	> 50 years of age or immunocompromised	Ceftriaxone -Plus- Vancomycin -Plus- Ampicillin
Healthcare-associated infectious diarrhea	*Clostridium difficile*	Mild-moderate infection	Metronidazole (oral)
		Severe infection	Vancomycin (oral) or Fidaxomicin
		Severe, complicated infection (e.g., ileus)	Vancomycin (oral) -Plus- Intravenous metronidazole
Community-acquired infectious diarrhea	*Shigella* *Salmonella* *Escherichia coli* *Campylobacter* *Clostridium difficile* (uncommon)	See above	Fluoroquinolone or TMP/SMX if antibiotic therapy is necessary

Index